Doctor–Patient Communication

Doctor–Patient Communication

Edited by

David Pendleton
*Royal College of General Practioners
London, U.K.*

and

John Hasler
*Regional Adviser in General Practice,
John Radcliffe Hospital
Oxford, U.K.*

1983

ACADEMIC PRESS
A Subsidiary of Harcourt Brace Jovanovich, Publishers
London   New York
Paris   San Diego   San Francisco   São Paulo
Sydney   Tokyo   Toronto

ACADEMIC PRESS INC. (LONDON) LTD.
24/28 Oval Road,
London NW1

United States Edition published by
ACADEMIC PRESS INC.
111 Fifth Avenue
New York, New York 10003

British Library Cataloguing in Publication Data
Doctor–Patient Communication.
  1. Physician and patient   2. Communication in medicine
I. Pendleton, D.   II. Hasler, J.
610.69'6   R727.3

ISBN 0–12–549880–2

LCCCN 82–73799

Typeset by Deltatype, Ellesmere Port
Printed and bound by T. J. Press (Padstow) Ltd.

Contributors

Michael Argyle: *Reader in Social Psychology, Department of Experimental Psychology, South Parks Road, University of Oxford, Oxford, U.K.*

Stephen Bochner: *Senior Lecturer, Department of Psychology, University of New South Wales, Australia.*

Ann Cartwright: *Director, Institute for Social Studies in Medical Care, 14 South Hill Park, Hampstead, London, NW3 2SB, U.K.*

Paul Freeling: *General Practitioner and Head, Unit of General Practice, St. George's Hospital Medical School, Cranmer Terrace, London, SW17, U.K.*

Muir Gray *Community Physician, Oxford District Community Health Officer, Radcliffe Infirmary, Woodstock Road, Oxford, U.K.*

John Hasler: *General Practitioner, Regional Adviser in General Practice, Oxford Region, Hon. Secretary of Council, Royal College of General Practitioners, 14 Princes Gate, Hyde Park, London SW7 1PU, U.K.*

Joseph Jaspars: *Lecturer in Psychology, Department of Experimental Psychology, University of Oxford and Fellow of St. Edmund Hall, Oxford, England.*

Jennifer King: *Social Psychologist, Department of Experimental Psychology, University of Oxord, South Parks Road, Oxford, U.K.*

Philip Ley: *Professor, Clinical Psychology Unit, University of Sydney, Australia.*

Marshall Marinker: *Director M.S.D. Foundation, Tavistock House, Tavistock Square, London, WC1H U.K.*

David Metcalfe: *General Practitioner, Professor, Department of General Practice, University of Manchester Medical School, Rusholme Health Centre, Walmer Street, Manchester M14 5NP, U.K.*

David Pendleton: *Stuart Fellow, Royal College of General Practitioners, 14 Princes Gate, Hyde Park, London, SW7 1PU, U.K.*

Peter Pritchard: *General Practitioner, Monks Corner, 31 Martins Lane, Dorchester On Thames, Oxfordshire, U.K.*

Theo Schofield: *General Practitioner, Associate Adviser in General Practice, Oxford Region, Postgraduate Office, Medical School Offices, John Radcliffe Hospital, Headington, Oxford, U.K.*

Peter Tate: *General Practitioner, Course Organiser in General Practice, Postgraduate Office, Medical School Offices, John Radcliffe Hospital, Headington, Oxford, U.K.*

Richard Wakeford: *Senior Research Associate, Office of the Regius Professor of Physic, Cambridge University School of Clinical Medicine, Cambridge, U.K.*

Preface

In this book the reader will find contributions by general practitioners and behavioural scientists. These are the two groups who have been most concerned with writing and researching on the subject of doctor–patient communication. All of those who have written chapters are interested in the subject and most might even be called enthusiasts. Inevitably, enthusiasm generates enthusiasm and it should not be surprising that several of the chapters represent some of the work of a group of colleagues from one particular part of the United Kingdom. All of the contributors, however, have published on this subject elsewhere.

The editors have in no way attempted to influence those who have written the essays to represent a particular point of view or even to use a common style of presentation. Each chapter is an essay which represents the views and reading of its author. Each chapter stands in its own right. The reader will, therefore, find it easy to browse through the book. It is not necessary for any reader to read the contributions from beginning to end. On the contrary, it is hoped that all readers will find a contribution which is provocative.

The book is intended as a resource for those who are teachers of medical students or experienced general practitioners. It is also intended for those applied behavioural scientists who find that an interest in communication leads them to investigate phenomena outside the laboratory. For this reason, each chapter contains references which will help the reader to follow-up the interests and themes delineated in its pages.

Finally, the editors would have found the book much less of a pleasure to produce had it not been for the help and supportive criticism of the following: the colleagues and friends of the Department of Experimental Psychology of the University of Oxford, the course organizers of the Oxford Vocational Training scheme in general practice and the Officers and staff of the Royal College of General Practitioners. In particular we should like to thank Barbara Vaughan, Ann McKendry, Valerie Mitchell and Judith Halliwell.

January 1983   David Pendleton and John Hasler

Contents

To Professor Patrick Byrne CBE, PRCGP

Introduction

David Pendleton and John Hasler

There are those who would argue that extensive doctor–patient communication is a luxury that few can afford. The pressures of patient demand do not allow the subject to be seen as anything more than a luxury which can easily be forfeited in the pursuit of accurate diagnoses and sound management of problems. This is an argument to which neither the editors nor the other contributors to this volume would subscribe for the reasons which we shall outline here.

In a recent study, a small but carefully selected sample of patients were asked about their experiences of medical care (Pendleton, 1981). The respondents were selected so that people from all social class groups, both sexes and a wide age range were represented in the study. They were asked about their worst and best experiences of medical care so that it was possible to deduce the factors which distinguished consultations the patients thought were "good" from those they thought were "bad". From this study, it became clear that, if the clinical decision making was faulty in an important way – if there was a wrong diagnosis made or inappropriate treatment was recommended – the patients described the consultation as a bad one. But in order for the consultation to be considered a good one, not only did the clinical medicine have to be of a high standard, but also the communication between the doctor and patient had to be satisfactory. The patients thus had two criteria for judging a consultation to be good. One criterion was good clinical decision making. The other was good communication which they described as the doctor listening well and volunteering information and explanations. They also said that they liked to be involved in the decisions which were made in the consultation. Patients spoke spontaneously of the importance of good communication with the doctor.

Ann Cartwright (Cartwright, 1967; Cartwright and Anderson, 1981) has demonstrated that patients express more dissatisfaction with the information they receive from doctors than with any other aspect of medical care. This is an important dimension of doctor–patient communication and is one which affects the patient's knowledge and understanding of health and how to protect it. Information given can also help patients to understand better the problem they have taken to the doctor for attention.

From these and other studies discussed in the subsequent chapters, we can see that doctor–patient communication is a concern of patients. What is more, it has been demonstrated that a substantial proportion of patients' anxieties about going to see the doctor are attributed by the patients to difficulties they anticipate in making matters clear to the doctor (Fitton and Acheson, 1979).

But it is not just patients who experience difficulties making matters clear. It has been demonstrated that 20–25% of consultations in general practice pose the doctors with communication difficulties (Pendleton, 1979). This may be the mere tip of an iceberg, moreover, since these were difficulties reported by the doctors themselves. In this study, the difficulties described by the doctors seemed to fall into two major categories. Eighty per cent of the problems were difficulties in the transmission of information whereas 13·5% of the problems arose when the doctor attempted to persuade the patient on a matter. (The literature on patient adherence to medical advice suggests that this may well be where the underestimate occurs. This evidence is considered later in Chapter 4.)

For doctors and patients alike, the experience of communication difficulties in general practice consultations suggests that the study of doctor–patient communication is an important one. It has, as the jargon would have it, a considerable degree of face validity.

Further evidence comes from research which has shown that even experienced medical practitioners may fail to diagnose problems accurately or to notice them at all due to poor or inadequate communication between the doctor and the patient (Maguire, 1981; Marks *et al.*, 1979). Thus, for purely clinical reasons, good communication is necessary. Future chapters will indicate that communication is implicated, not only in the outcomes of medical care but also in the patients' decision to use medical services. Some have even suggested that the increasing burden of malpractice litigation in the United States may be put down to poor communication between the consumers and providers of the medical services (Bay, 1975).

There has certainly been an increase in the attention paid to doctor–patient communication by the social science fraternity in recent years. Any representative survey of the relevant literature will show that the number of publications on the subject has been steadily rising since the 1960s. The 1970s saw a virtual explosion in the published work. In addition, the number of symposia, conferences, workshops and other academic meetings concerned with the topic has mirrored the expansion in the literature. The original impetus for this volume came from one such meeting although this book has grown considerably in the subsequent months.

In the first chapter, David Pendleton surveys the extensive literature on doctor–patient communication up to the writing of this book. He provides a model which enables the literature to be organized around the event of the consultation itself. The book is then divided into four major sections.

In Part I, Michael Argyle relates the work on social skills and social skills training to the practice of medicine and Peter Tate discusses the related matter of doctors' styles in the consultation. These contributions concern the behaviour to be seen in the consultation.

In Part II, four essays provide an insight into some of the psychological perspectives on the consultation. Philip Ley summarizes much of his own work and that of others to account for some of the important failures of communication to be found in medical practice. Jennifer King describes the importance of patients' beliefs about their health and relates these to the processes and outcomes of medical care. Stephen Bochner relates the doctor's and the patient's behaviour to their respective professional and lay cultures. In so doing, Bochner reminds the observer that behaviour cannot be understood adequately if it is removed from its cultural context. Jaspars and colleagues describe the ways in which academic social psychology attempts to study behaviour in the consulting room. In addition, the authors provide an account of other useful psychological contributions to understanding doctors' and patients' behaviour, namely attribution theory and the work on locus of control.

The doctor–patient relationship is another context in which communication takes place and this is the subject of Part III of the book. Paul Freeling argues persuasively that the relationship provides an additional resource for the medical practitioner but one which is not always easy to use. Ann Cartwright asserts that prescribing may be used as a substitute for adequate communication and may, therefore, prevent the relationship from being used to good effect. Muir Gray draws on his considerable experience of dealing with elderly people in the community. He reminds us that communication does not only take place in the consulting room but also in the patient's home and relates some of the problems which can arise in this setting. Peter Pritchard, on the other hand, would have us remember that communication does not just take place between a doctor and a patient. In describing the growth of the Patient Participation movement, he shows how the relationship between a doctor and his practice population may be developed and may promote a greater involvement in the running of the practice and in thinking about health matters.

If all of this attention to the subject of doctor–patient communication is to make any difference to medical practice, it has to influence medical education at some level. Part IV considers this matter. David Metcalfe, who has devoted many years to undergraduate medical education, argues that there are important ways in which undergraduate medical education is incompatible with medical practice. Richard Wakeford goes on to describe the attempts being made to help medical students learn to communicate with patients more effectively and to prevent the deterioration of communication skills described by some authors. John Hasler and Theo Schofield each consider the impact of communication skills training at the postgraduate, vocational training level.

In Part V, the concluding chapter, Marshall Marinker looks to the future and recommends that the application of peer evaluation and video-technology might be developed in continuing medical education. He also argues that the liaison between medical practitioners and behavioural scientists must continue and increase.

This volume is neither a textbook nor a practical guide. It is a collection of essays on an important subject. The contributions represent the breadth of thinking and variety of approaches to be found in the literature on doctor–patient communication. It is hoped that teachers, researchers and general practitioners will find the essays helpful, informative and provocative.

REFERENCES

Bay, J. C. (1975). Communications the key. *Mich. Med.* **74** (15), 299.
Cartwright, A. (1967). *Patients and their Doctors*. Atherton, N.Y.
Cartwright, A. and Anderson, R. (1981). *General practice revisited*. Tavistock Publications, London.
Fitton, F. and Acheson, H. W. K. (1979). *The Doctor–Patient Relationship*. H.M.S.O., London.
Maguire, P. (1981). Doctor–patient skills. In *Social Skills and Health* (J. M. Argyle, ed.). Methuen, London.
Marks, J. N., Goldberg, D. P. and Hillier, V. (1979). Determinants of the ability of general practitioners to detect psychiatric illness. *Psychol. Med.* **9**, 337–353.
Pendleton, D. A. (1979). Assessing the communication difficulty in general practice consultations. In *Research in Psychology and Medicine* Vol. II (D. J. Oborne, M. M. Gruneberg and J. R. Eiser, eds). Academic Press, London.
Pendleton, D. A. (1981). *Doctor–Patient Communication*. Unpublished doctoral dissertation, University of Oxford.

1 Doctor–Patient Communication: A Review

David Pendleton

1 INTRODUCTION

1.1 Model

Research into complex phenomena is inevitably fragmented since no individual study can hope to be exhaustive. The study of doctor–patient communication is a complex phenomenon in this sense but the matter is made even more fragmented since no model or theory exists which would integrate the studies. Even if such a model were devised, the residual differences of approach, of definitions of key terms, of methodology and of aims might prove impossibly confusing. The purpose of this chapter is to consider the major approaches to the study of doctor–patient communication and to propose a means by which the studies can be classified. Rieker and Begun (1980) have provided a social model of the illness process, but a model will be proposed, which will serve to locate most of the studies of doctor–patient communication and its associated issues. The model (Fig 1.1) shows the place of the primary care consultation in the cycle of primary medical care but it would serve equally well for any patient initiated medical consultation.

It will be argued in subsequent sections that a more systematic approach is required in the doctor–patient literature. Those variables should be considered together which constitute input to the consultation. These are factors which may influence the way the consultation is conducted. They may include attributes of doctor and patient, aspects of the patient's condition, features of the surgery and so on. On the other hand, variables which are outcomes from consultations should also, logically, be considered together. Outcomes, we

DOCTOR   PATIENT

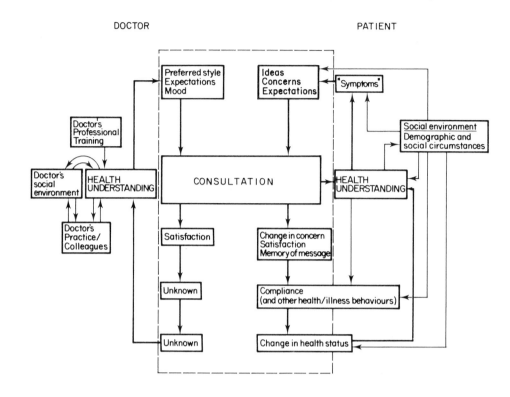

shall see, may affect doctor and patient in a variety of ways and over a broad span of time. The consultation's processes, it will be argued, can only be understood adequately in the context of input and outcome. Without these twin anchors, the study of consultation processes will lack any adequate criterion or appropriateness. If, for example, any scheme for describing consultation processes is to be chosen, the criteria for choice of scheme would include the proportion of variance in outcomes the description explains (see Section 5.1 on process and outcomes.) Without this criterion, it may be impossible to choose between descriptive schemes other than on grounds of elegance or expedience.

In the model proposed, the patient is placed in the context of his demographic and social circumstances which would include his home and family. This environment plays a part in determining some of the relevant psychological characteristics of the patient but, as Argyle *et al.* (1981b) point out, this relationship of person to situation may well be reciprocal. Not only do situations or circumstances influence the people in them but the people both choose and influence their circumstances. The relevant psychological characteristics of the patient in this case would include their health beliefs, their locus of control and broader attributions. These have been shown to influence a patient's "health behaviour" to a far greater extent than more global personality variables such as introversion-extraversion (Becker *et al.*, 1977; Becker, 1979). These psychological characteristics are also more predictive of an individual's health behaviour than their demographic and social position *per se* (see Chapter 5, this volume). The model suggests, therefore, that the patient's broader social circumstances affect consultations primarily through their influence on his health beliefs, locus of control and broader attributions. The patient's attitudes and beliefs about health, illness and medical treatment, I shall call his *health understanding*. These determine the ways in which changes in bodily states and psychological states are perceived (Kasl, 1974; Zola, 1972). They may not be registered at all but if any significance is attributed to them then it will be against the background of, indeed, to some extent, determined by the patient's health understanding (Pennebaker and Skelton, 1981). Differences in the perception of symptoms certainly "resist being reformulated as simply one or another of the Health Belief Model variables" (Kasl, 1974, p. 448).

The perception of a symptom *qua* symptom will then require that a choice is made between three possibilities: to do nothing, to treat it oneself, or to seek help. In this choice, one's social environment plays a significant role. Zola (1972) has reviewed the considerable literature on this decision making process and has emphasized the importance of the lay referral and support functions of one's social environment. The likelihood of deciding to visit the doctor is therefore crudely conceived of as a function of: (i) previous history of visits to the doctor, (ii) social environment in the form of lay referral and support systems, (iii) degree of concern and expectations about the problem and its treatment, derived from (iv) health beliefs and attributional biases.

When the patient approaches the consulting room, therefore, his degree of concern about his symptoms will be the most salient and pressing aspect of his health understanding.

To locate the patient's health understanding at this point allows for it to be influenced by the patient's social situation. It allows for the understanding to play a part in the decision to seek medical help and in the patient's input to the consultation. Finally, it allows for doctor–patient contact to influence *health understanding*. This may be either direct influence in the consultation by way of specific health education or indirect influence as the patient observes the changes in his health status as a result of the consultation and treatment.

This takes into consideration the omissions in the Health Belief Model summarized by Kasl (1974). He pointed out that the HBM leaves out:

(1) The patient's social environment which therefore omits lay referral and social support.

(2) The doctor–patient interaction about which he states: "In short, the Health Belief Model variables do not operate in a vacuum but in specific settings of which the doctor–patient relationship is a crucial one" (p. 447).

(3) Perceptions of symptoms and lay constructions of illness and the sick role. Here he singles out social representations as a relevant behavioural science concept but a more helpful reference would have been to the literature on attributions of causality and on locus of control which broaden his emphasis considerably (see Chapter 7, this volume).

All of this allows an input – process – outcome formulation of the consultation to be made similar to Donabedian's (1967) structure, process, outcome model. The patient presents to the doctor with one or more symptoms plus an understanding or theory about the symptom(s) which has given rise to sufficient concern for the appointment to have been made. Thus the symptoms, the patient's ideas and concern about them and, to some extent, his expectations form the input to the consultation and collectively constitute the problem(s) in hand.

1.2 Interaction Between Doctor and Patient

The consultation itself forms an opportunity for doctor and patient to influence each other in identifying and choosing the appropriate actions for each problem presented. In this endeavour a variety of consulting strategies may be adopted by either party. The more often certain blends of behaviours are repeated between consultations, the more a style of consulting may be said to exist. Byrne and Long (1976), for example, have identified seven styles of doctor behaviour which range from doctor centred to patient centred. These styles are said to be adopted by most doctors and maintained with little variation between consultations. We shall come to see, however, that empirical quantitative attempts to describe doctor's styles have been elusive.

It is in the consultation that attempts to modify both the symptoms and the health understanding of the patient can be made. The patient may even be persuaded to change his behaviour in order to live a more healthy life. Attempts to describe consultation processes are of three kinds: quantitative, qualitative and evaluative. Each of these is described in detail elsewhere but the model suggests that the outcomes of any consultation are a function of its inputs and its processes.

The outcomes of consultations, like their inputs and processes, may be physical and/or psychological in a social context. Moreover, the outcomes may be immediate, intermediate or long term. In the literature on the consultation these distinctions in both quality and time scale of outcomes have been blurred but it will help considerably to maintain the distinctions. Immediate outcomes from the consultation, so far as the patient is concerned, would include the patient's satisfaction with the consultation, his memory for the doctor's explanations and instructions and changes in the patient's concern about his problem. The changes may be in either direction or the concern may not have been influenced at all, e.g. when a referral to a consultant has been made. Intermediate outcomes from the consultation include the much investigated phenomenon of compliance with the doctor's instructions. It should be noted, however, that as soon as a patient has left the consulting room, the influence of the social environment and health understanding continue to act on the patient and the influence of the doctor will begin to wane. The doctor is usually heavily weighted in the equation of influences, however, and he may also have taken an opportunity to educate the patient's health understanding. Nevertheless, the investigation of compliance incorporates a number of uncontrolled and uncontrollable variables which will account for variance. For this reason, it will be argued, researchers would do well to investigate immediate outcomes first.

The long-term outcome of greatest importance is a change in the health status of the patient. This is rarely reported in the literature. The reasons for this are several but the range of problems presented in general practice in the U.K. is one reason. Many of the problems are self-limiting and, therefore, recovery would have been spontaneous if the problem were to have remained untreated. Changes in the patient's health understanding, which are contingent upon spontaneous remission of symptoms, may well be superstitious. What is more, other problems presented to the G.P. may be psychological or social in aetiology and highly complex in nature so that changes may take years to achieve. More importantly, a large proportion of G.P.s' workload is made up of consultations in which the doctor has the pleasure of reassuring the patient that nothing is wrong with him at all. General practitioners in this country have made a concern for health rather than sickness their legitimate aim (RCGP, 1972) so no change in health status would be registered, although a small change should have been detectable in his health understanding and concern.

Changes in health status have been, and are continuing to be, investigated although more usually in hospital clinics than in primary care (Britton *et al.*, 1980). An equally profitable long-term outcome to be investigated, the model suggests, would be long-term changes in the patient's understanding. The literature on Health Beliefs (see Chapter 5, this volume) is replete with studies on changes in those aspects of health understanding. The literature on health locus of control recommends itself as an outcome measure, but it is long-term changes in the patient's health understanding as a whole which will form the strongest influence on the patient's health behaviour in his social setting.

Finally, on the patient's side, the model makes clear the role of its various elements in the repeated *cycle* of continuing primary care which is the usual pattern in the U.K.

What has yet to be explained, however, is that the issue of the doctor–patient relationship and the matter of faith in the doctor as a healer is also a part of what we have called the patient's health understanding since it cannot logically be separated from the issue of "perceived effectiveness of treatment" in the Health Belief Model and the role of "powerful others" in the health locus of control literature. In this way the doctor–patient relationship plays its part in the decision to visit the doctor and is also modified by each consultation.

The preceding discussion of the model has been largely concerned with the patient. This is an accurate reflection of the literature. A few studies have examined the issue of what frustrates doctors in their consultations (Cartwright and Anderson, 1979, 1981; Mechanic, 1974) but these studies have largely been remote from actual consultations, depending on the doctor's memory over a considerable time span. Bennett *et al.* (1978) conducted a study in which types of problems and types of patients had to be rated by their sample of general practitioners, but this study too is of uncertain validity due to the possible distortions which memory might effect. Melville (1980a) has demonstrated that job satisfaction expressed by general practitioners is associated with their prescribing patterns. Job satisfaction is slow to change and is influenced by many things other than just consultations. Job satisfaction is also related to the extent to which general practitioners perceive problems presented to them as trivial (Mechanic, 1974). Other related variables were the doctor's social orientation to medicine, the number of patients the doctor saw each day (the more consultations, the greater the proportion seen as trivial), and his age at entry to medical school – the older at entry, the more consultations were seen as trivial. This attitude to triviality was also investigated by Gough (1977). Gough concluded that the doctor who saw complaints as trivial would be older at entry to medical school, more able at scientific thinking, of affiliative temperament, non-conforming or unconventional in methods of seeking academic or intellectual goals, better prepared in pre-medical subjects and somewhat inclined to think psychologically or intuitively about himself or others.

A tendency to be authoritarian characterizes some doctors' consulting style and Lloyd (1974) saw this as unremarkable but recommended that something be done to change this attitude in order to meet community needs.

Doctors' attitudes are, to some extent, influenced by their professional training, their work setting and colleagues. It is likely that their conception of the rules which should operate in consultations will also derive in part from these sources, whereas consultations' norms can only be established in the consultations. It is also likely that consultations will play their part in modifying a doctor's attitudes, job satisfaction and the rules followed just as these influence the doctor's consultations. It is unfortunate, however, that little evidence exists which would help us to complete the model from the doctor's point of view. Much exists in the way of opinion from informed sources but empirical work is needed which will help us to understand how differences in the ways specific doctors approach specific consultations affect the process of the consultation and its outcomes.

There is considerable information available, by contrast, on the differences in doctors' behaviour in specific consultations and how these are related to outcomes in the patients. This leaves much of the doctors' behaviour inadequately grounded in the doctors *per se*. We know more of how doctors perceive patients than we know of how they perceive themselves, and this leaves unanswered questions regarding how doctors approach and emerge from their consultations. The relevant literature on consultation processes is dealt with under the appropriate headings below (see Sections 2.2, 3 and 5). Where studies are available or where matters are covered in this book, an entry is made in the model under the "doctor" heading.

In summary, the model is based on the available literature and is used to structure the remaining sections of this chapter.

2 INPUT TO THE CONSULTATION

The relevant antecedents to consultations may influence, to an extent still to be determined, the content of the consultation. These will be referred to, collectively, as the consultation's input. This section will consider the relevant aspects, how they have been described and the extent of their influence on consultation processes and outcomes.

2.1 Input Alone

Most studies of inputs to consultations also attempt to show how these affect consultation processes. One clear exception is that of Bruhn and Trevino (1979) who have examined patients' perceptions of their health needs. They identified four kinds of health needs which logically will constitute inputs to a consultation.

(1) The patient's *present health status* needs to be made clear by the doctor.
(2) The patient needs *knowledge* about related health matters.
(3) The patient may need *treatment*.
(4) The patient needs *support*.

The authors devised a 30 item forced binary choice questionnaire to assess these health needs and recommended its use by physicians in their first encounter with patients. They maintained that compliance is dependent on the bond between physician and patient. They further maintained that this bond is strengthened when doctors' and patients' needs are complementary. They quoted some evidence for these assertions but these *empirical* issues remained untested in their paper.

In addition, Krantz *et al.* (1980) have devised the Krantz Health Opinion Survey which measures the extent to which patients would like information and would like to be involved in their medical care.

McKinlay (1975) by contrast, examined the levels of comprehension of frequently used medical terms in a sample of 87 unskilled working class mothers in Scotland. His sample was divided into two sub-samples of "utilizers and under-utilizers" of maternity services who were interviewed four times over an 18 month period. He found that there was a significantly higher level of comprehension in the "utilizers" compared with the "under-utilizers". Among the utilizers, there was a slightly higher level of comprehension in mothers with more than one child rather than first time mothers but the most significant finding for the present discussion is that the doctors of the women in the study markedly and consistently underestimated their levels of comprehension.

Coope and Metcalfe (1979) administered a ten question multiple choice questionnaire about personal preventive medicine, treatment and the use of health services to 664 patients in doctors' waiting rooms. They reported a clear trend between social class and amount of knowledge—the higher the patient's social class, the more they knew. They also reported what they called "a distressing degree of ignorance on some topics", for example, only approximately 10% of the patients in the study were aware of the possibility that antibiotics might lead to diarrhoea as a side effect. There was slight evidence that women knew more than men and that knowledge was especially poor in males over 39 from social classes 4 and 5.

2.2 Input and Consultation Processes

This section concerns studies which attempt to show how the consultation's processes are affected largely by attributes of physician or patient which affect their behaviour.

Zola (1963) showed that patient and physician attributes as well as the clinic's spatial design and organization affected doctor–patient communication, diagnosis and patient care. He showed that diagnoses varied regarding psychosocial problems according to the patient's ethnic background when similar symptoms were described. He showed that doctors from some medical specialities were more likely than those from other specialities to ignore psychosocial problems and that clinic design and organization can act as a barrier or as a stimulus to communication. This was a study which would benefit from experimental replication in a British general practice setting since we do not know whether the "similar" symptoms, for example, were sufficiently different for different diagnoses to be legitimate. We also do not know whether the epidemiology of different medical specialities would explain their likelihood of dealing with psychosocial problems, or whether this finding is indicative of attitudinal differences or even whether psychosocial problems are considered beyond the scope of the specialities investigated.

Zola's attempts to study input-process associations initiated an interest in these matters which was slow to develop, but studies in the 1970s have shown an increasing sophistication in approach. De Boer (1973) reported a series of studies with colleagues in Holland, which showed that changes in a GP's attitudes to psychological problems were associated with an increasing ability to deal with these problems in role-played consultations. Similarly Melville (1980b) investigated the repeat prescribing of psychotropic drugs and concluded that "the treatment of patients with repeat prescriptions for Librium and Valium reflects the doctor's attitudes more than the patient's condition" (p. 113). She conducted a path analysis in support of this contention which accounted for 58% of the variance in the dependent measure. Stewart and Buck (1977) studied the extent to which a group of five family doctors in a Canadian group practice, were aware of and responded to the problems of a sample of 299 of their patients. The patients were interviewed before they saw the doctor and were followed up for three months. They demonstrated that their doctors had a high percentage of perfect scores on knowledge of the patients' discomfort, worry and disturbances to their daily living but a low percentage of perfect scores on knowledge of their patients' social problems. The doctors, additionally, had made successful attempts to deal with their patients' discomfort but had either ignored or been unsuccessful with their patients' worry, disturbance to daily living and social problems. There was, finally, a low but significant positive correlation between knowledge and response for all four types of problem.

Browne (1978) provided evidence that some patients in her North American study may have taught physicians to avoid the task in consultations so that they did not actually get well. She found that instances of the patient avoiding the task when the doctor approached it and the patient's positive response to the doctor's avoiding the task were significantly more frequent among patients who were "dysfunctional" (unwell), psychologically distressed and frequent attenders. Whereas, mutual approach towards the task of getting the patient well by both doctor and patient was significantly related to patients who were "functionally healthy", not psychologically distressed and infrequent attenders. This complicity in task avoidance was pointed out much earlier by Balint (1964) but was not investigated empirically by him.

Raynes (1980) investigated which of a general practitioner's activities can be classed as routines and which are responsive to differences in the patient's presenting symptoms. Her U.K. sample was of ten G.P.s of whom she recorded one in three consultations in two morning and two evening surgeries. She examined the doctors' use of the following three "search procedures" and four patient management techniques:

(1) The G.P.'s questions: physical, social, emotional or administrative.
(2) The G.P.'s use of a physical examination.
(3) The G.P.'s use of the patient's notes.
(4) The G.P.'s prescribing practices (psychotropic or not).
(5) The G.P.'s referral of patients for evaluation or treatment.
(6) The G.P.'s recall of patients.
(7) The G.P.'s writing of certificates.

She classified the presenting symptoms into nine categories and analysed the frequency of the seven activities in two rather different types of consultations, namely, predominantly physical versus predominantly psychosocial consultations. She demonstrated that types of questioning and the use of psychotropic prescribing were responsive to change whereas the other five activities were not—they were more ritualistic. Unfortunately, this study is marred by poor statistics and design. First, there were only 19 psychosocial consultations whereas there were ten doctors and we are not told the distribution of these 19 cases between the doctors. Secondly, analysis of variance or discriminant analysis would possibly have been a more helpful procedure since this would have enabled the relative effects of type of problem, doctor and attributes of the patient or consultation to have been treated simultaneously.

More directly in the Zola tradition, Rhee (1977) attempted to determine the relative importance of the physician's personal and situational characteristics in the quality of patient care. He studied 454 doctors who discharged 2517 patients from 22 short-term general hospitals in Hawaii in 1968. He considered as independent variables: the extent of the doctor's specialization, their type of medical school and their number of years in practice. He also analysed their type of outpatient clinic and the type of hospital in which they worked. The dependent measure was the physician's performance judged against standards set by 15 doctors. This was called the physician performance index or PPI. He reported that the following results were found:

(1) The doctors' present work environment had more influence on the quality of care (PPI score) than their formal medical training, viz. the situation was more influential than what the doctors had internalized.

(2) The organizational influence decreased with more doctor training.

(3) The hospital work settings had distinct attributes which influenced the behaviour of doctors independently of doctors' qualifications.)

This study demonstrates, however, a central problem with research of this kind, namely, that the distribution of doctors and settings is not random. Argyle's *et al.* (1981b) comments are again relevant here since, to some extent, doctors choose the settings in which they work, influence those settings and choose new doctors for them. The influence of the setting is, to some extent, an artefact of the influence of the people within them. To this extent the situational influence is essentially interpersonal in nature, but this does suggest that the traditional idea of a doctor who is trained to respond to predefined conditions in prescribed ways, does not explain adequately variations in quality of care.

The literature on the issue of locus of control is considered elsewhere (see Chapter 7, this volume) but the simple finding of relevance here is that patients who are high on internal locus of control seek much more information in consultations than those who are external controllers (Wallston *et al.*, 1974; Wallston and Wallston, 1978). Thus it could be argued that the situational influence on the doctor includes the patient's behaviour. Naturally, the literature on giving and receiving of medical information is more complex than this. Boreham and Gibson (1978) consider much of the relevant work in the introduction to their study, which was designed to discover how much information was offered by the doctor and how much was requested by the patient. Their semi-random sample of 80 consultations was made up of 20 randomly selected from each of four doctors who had been selected by personal contact with the researchers. The study was conducted in Queensland, Australia. Four research instruments were used:

(1) A brief questionnaire to the doctors which asked what sorts of information, in general, patients should obtain during consultations. It also asked what is desirable and undesirable patient behaviour.

(2) An interview of patients before the consultation. This examined three areas: attitudes of the patient towards gaining knowledge about their problem and its treatment; the extent of their present knowledge; and their feelings about what is desirable patient behaviour.

(3) Details of the patient's illness/problem were taken from the doctors' notes.

(4) An analysis (by one of the researchers sitting in on the consultation) of the interaction between doctor and patient. This divided the interview into four areas: (i) initial discussion of symptoms or reasons for the visit; (ii) the medical examination; (iii) the establishment of the diagnosis; (iv) the prescription of treatment.

Of particular interest here were those aspects of the consultation wherein information was supplied to patients about diagnosis and treatment and the number and type of questions the patient asked. The scheme for scoring the communication of information concerning the illness was (1) diagnosis only, (2) minimal explanation, (3) detailed explanation, (4) whether the condition had worsened or improved, (5) aetiology, (6) what to expect in the way of further symptoms. Information concerning the treatment was scored: (1) "blue pills", (2) name of drug, (3) type of drug, (4) effect of drug, (5) side effects of drug, (6) instructions for the patient.

Boreham and Gibson report finding the following:

(1) There was sufficient difference in the way initial and follow-up consultations were run for them to have to split their data this way.

(2) Information about diagnosis was usually given in the patient's initial consultation and was rarely asked for by the patient. Few patients questioned the doctor on any of the six issues about the diagnosis, so that what they were told depended, largely, on what the doctor offered. The doctors answered what they were asked in all but one case.

(3) Information about treatment was rarely asked for by the patient so that, again, what the patient was told depended, largely, on what the doctor offered. Only in 1-in-2 initial consultations and 1-in-4 follow-up consultations did patients ask questions about treatment other than the name of the drug. Little information was offered by the doctor about drug side effects.

Boreham and Gibson concluded that there was little evidence that doctors manipulated to achieve the dominant position (in contrast to Stimson and Webb, 1975) but much more support for the notion that patients tended to think that questioning the doctor implied lack of confidence (Coe, 1970). Patients express a desire for information prior to consultations but when it is not offered it is not asked for, despite the fact that the doctors almost always gave it when requested. They also found that the doctors' and the patients' views about what constituted a "good" patient were similar—viz. essentially passive and deferential. A similar finding was that of Pratt *et al.* (1957) who pointed out that patients appeared to wait for the doctor to take the initiative in explanations whereas the doctor perceived the patient's lack of enquiry as indicating uninterest or incompetence to understand.

In order to explain deference, or even apparent diffidence in the consultation, one has to examine input variables. Cartwright and O'Brien (1976) resorted to the notion of social distance brought about by differences in social class between doctor and patient. The prediction can, therefore, be tested that, the greater the social distance, the more likely an individual is to be diffident in the presence of the higher status other. Another possible explanation would be that the more worried a patient is, the more he needs to perceive the doctor as a powerful person. This may work as a linear relationship or as a curvilinear relationship. In the former case, the more concerned the patient, the fewer questions he would ask. In the latter, there would be an increase in question asking as concern increases to a certain level, after which higher concern would be associated with a decreasing number of questions.

One final possibility is that, if the doctor acts as an essential healing agent, then the patient would not need to ask many questions, nor even, for that matter, to comply very closely with the advice given. This idea (Balint, 1964) does not lend itself readily to investigation, since its prediction is general. The closest one might come in this matter would be to examine the statements of satisfaction offered by the patient about the consultation. In those cases in which concern is reduced, the higher the patient's initial concern, the greater the proportion of statements they would offer about the doctor as a person as against other aspects of the consultation such as the treatment given, the information offered or the explanations given.

2.3 Conclusions

The investigation of antecedents to the consultation has drawn attention to both similarities and differences between patients. Similarities, however, are usually much less informative than differences. The measurement of differences between patients produces variation and this can be used subsequently to discover those things with which covariation occurs. To show, for example, that patients differed in their medical knowledge enabled Coope and Metcalfe (1979) to demonstrate that these differences followed social class lines—that is, that social class covaried with medical knowledge. But in order to apply this kind of research, antecedents must be identified which covary with other measures which can be influenced in some way. Browne's (1978) finding that frequent attenders were more likely to engage in task avoidance in the consultation implied that compensatory action might be taken by the doctor. What is more, the significance of findings which do not influence subsequent behaviour in any demonstrable way is hard to judge. Thus, the identification of differences between patients in antecedents to the consultation invites, and, to some extent, requires the investigation of related consultation processes. This argument can be carried further, however, since it is generally the outcomes from consultations which most practitioners seek to influence and this suggests that even in the investigation of antecedents, their effect on process and outcome is of particular relevance.

3 CONSULTATION PROCESSES

This section deals with studies on consultation processes *per se* which have made little or no attempt to relate their findings to input or outcome. There have been five approaches: sociolinguistic, non-verbal, clinical, verbal content and evaluative. It will be argued, at the end of this section, that these process descriptions, which lack any explicit relationship to input or outcome variables, may be of dubious validity.

3.1 The Sociolinguistic Approach

Sociolinguistic studies are concerned with the language used by doctor and patient and they attempt to categorize each utterance into types. Skopek (1979) and Cassell *et al.* (1977) identified eight different *types* of utterance which they called main conversational divisions. These were:

(1) Opening/closing—primarily concerned with greetings and endings of consultations.

(2) Narrative—sequences reporting on facts, symptoms and events.

(3) Explanation—the giving of reasons.

(4) Interrogation—questions and answers.

(5) Elicitation—short questions to clarify a specific point.

(6) Bantering—casual joking on non-medical matters.

(7) Idling—casual conversation on non-medical matters.

(8) Discussing—presentation and consideration of a variety of matters relevant to the problem(s).

Conversation categorized into these types of utterance, they maintained, can also be analysed separately into a series of levels on which verbal communication occurs and at which communication problems arise. The *levels* they described were:

(1) "Acoustic"—sounds must be heard.

(2) "Phonological"—sounds must form recognizable words.

(3) "Syntactic"—words must form recognizable sentences.

(4) "Lexical"—words used must have recognizable meanings.

These first four levels are basic language requirements but more complex communication problems are associated with the final three levels:

(5) "Conceptual"—the knowledge and conceptions which govern the relevant subject matter, e.g. medical concepts. It is also to be noted that personal meanings evolve which doctor and patient may not share.

(6) "Intent"—the force, emphasis or importance associated with an issue and how it is perceived.

(7) "Credence"—the credibility of the utterance.

In the literature on doctor–patient communication, there exist almost as many schemes to describe the interaction as there are studies. The basic distinctions to be maintained, however, are relatively few. Types of utterance are certainly to be distinguished from levels of communication in the way described. Ford (1977) divides communication problems between doctor and patient into two basic kinds: problems of the communication channel, which vary from foreign language speakers to differences in popular usage of words, and more fundamental problems which "surface through the communication channel", such as differences in underlying assumptions, knowledge, attitudes and emotional needs (see also Crystal, 1976).

Sociolinguistic analysis of this kind also gives rise to studies which attempt to infer the rules of interaction which appear to underlie the consistencies in the interaction. Litton-Hawes (1978) studied 16 consultations and derived rules from the speaking turns. It was pointed out that the rules were asymmetrical in that each party did not follow the same rules. Examples of the rules thus generated were:

(1) If the doctor asks about a topic (X), the patient is obligated to imply (X).

(2) If the doctor asks about (X), the patients may ask a question about (X) before answering the doctor's question.

(3) Patients may imply new topics only after commenting on the topic implied in the doctor's previous turn.

(4) If the patient implies a new topic, the doctor is not obligated to comment on the topic.

This approach is painstaking and extremely expensive in terms of the time required and yet Frankel (1980) described how to conduct such microanalysis before describing the interactional rules he had derived from his extensive microanalysis of video-tape data. His rules included those relating to the organization of verbal and non-verbal behaviour and these were said to become salient within episodes of the consultation such as the history taking or the physical examination. An example of how this works is as follows. It was noticed that just prior to the point at which the doctor touches the patient's body in a physical examination, the doctor often starts to talk about something unrelated to the problem. This has the effect of shifting the patient's gaze from the approaching hands towards the doctor's face. Thus, the voice takes preference, according to Frankel, over touch in competing for visual attention. He then formulated this relationship into a rule:

> . . . in the presence of question formatted conversational object one should, as part of formulating a response shift, gaze toward the direction of the interlocutor prior to the end of a response which terminates a Q-A sequence. (Frankel: personal communication.)

This example from Frankel demonstrates how rules are "derived" from studying the minutiae of interaction. It also demonstrates some of the dangers of rules derived this way. It may be that the patient would look away from approaching hands out of fear or out of embarrassment. It may also be that the rule thus formulated is more complicated to understand than the original acts, but much of the work in this tradition follows the pattern described. Collett (1979) has distinguished between behaving according to rules and being aware of the rule. Observations made may demonstrate regularities but one may wish to question whether these imply the existence of rules since rules are usually associated with what is permissible and carry the implication of sanctions for rule breaking.

Coulthard and Ashby (1975) have taken this inferential approach one stage further by deriving an understanding of the *roles* occupied by the participants. They presented data from 24 consultations to show how the doctor directed the interviews to get the information he required. The roles they described were subsumed under the following two headings:

(1) Initiating and responding roles. Largely, it was the doctor who initiated and the patient who responded and these roles were maintained even when the patient attempted to initiate.

(2) Informant and recipient roles. Usually the doctor received information from the informing patient.

The limitations of this approach to doctor–patient communication are, first, that the cost of analysing minutiae is so high that usually sample sizes are small in sociolinguistic studies so that there may be difficulty in generalizing from the findings. Secondly, we are still relatively unsophisticated in analysing interaction—that is, in making the analysis genuinely interactional (Marsden, 1971). Thirdly, we are left to infer to a large extent. In one taxonomy for describing the doctor's and patient's verbal behaviour (Stiles, 1978), it is required that both form and intent of the utterance be coded and intention may only be inferred, but there exist difficulties in the over dependence on inference in the studies. Description can be relatively precise (although the validity of the categories chosen is usually left undiscussed) but the inference of intent as well as of rules and roles from consistencies noted leaves room for significant influence of the investigator. For these reasons, the rule's appropriateness should be tested by making it the basis of a hypothesis.

3.2 The Non-verbal Behaviour Approach

Boranic's (1979) assertion that non-verbal behaviour is not open to investigation, although it is a crucial element of medical consultations, was based upon the assumption that the investigation should be introspective. In this case, he argues, the perceiver's mind cannot be both the subject and the investigator. The literature on the role of non-verbal processes in the consultation has not made the introspective assumption, however, but has proceeded in a more orthodox way, borrowing many of its techniques and arguments from the considerable literature on non-verbal communication in social psychology. Strictly speaking, information gained about a patient's physical condition from a physical examination is both informative and behavioural and in this sense could be considered as non-verbal communication but more usually this view is not taken and non-verbal communication is seen to involve the transmission of messages between participants without words. This transmission may not be intended or may be misperceived but certainly social meaning may be communicated non-verbally (Birdwhistell, 1952). The main sub-divisions of non-verbal behaviour are: bodily contact, proximity, posture, physical appearance, facial and gestural movements, direction of gaze and the non-verbal aspects of speech—timing, emotional tone (pitch and stress), speech errors and accent (Argyle, 1969).

A number of authors have attempted to explain the relevance of non-verbal behaviour for a medical readership (Pietroni, 1976; Friedman, 1979), and they have included *olfaction* in the list of non-verbal sources of information since "some illnesses and treatments may act directly to produce unpleasant odours in the patient" (Friedman, 1979, p. 92).

The ability accurately to perceive a patient's emotional state is clearly one which doctors require in their daily work and most of the information about emotional state is transmitted non-verbally, especially through *facial expressions* and *tone of voice* (Argyle, 1975; Ekman *et al.*, 1972). It is also the case that patients are unusually receptive to the non-verbal behaviour of medical personnel, looking to them for cues as to how they ought to be feeling (Ellsworth *et al.*, 1978) especially since patients often feel that doctors may be withholding information from them for a variety of reasons (Cartwright, 1964) or that questioning the doctor may imply a lack of confidence in him (Coe, 1970), or just that the "good patient" should not question this busy, high status doctor (Taylor, 1979).

Patients' non-verbal expressiveness serves functions beyond the communication of emotions. *Non-verbal expression of symptoms* may be more accurate than verbal expression. Patients are often remarkably ignorant of the location and size of organs in the body and therefore their verbal descriptions cannot automatically be believed. There is also a guardedness or even embarrassment which accompanies descriptions of genital problems and this often produces a series of more or less comprehensible euphemisms for the doctor to disentangle. Additionally, some words have a meaning in popular language which have quite another meaning in medicine. Such a word is "stomach", for example, which means a particular body part to the doctor but means to the patient anywhere in the middle third of the trunk. Thus, doctors may form more accurate impressions of the location and spread of a problem by observing its non-verbal description (Miller, 1978).

The quality of an experience is also transmitted non-verbally. Verbal descriptions of pain can be confusing since we are not sure that a pain described as "stabbing" to one person would not be similar to one described as "sudden" to another. The distress experienced by the pain, however, is often communicated in its non-verbal description and this provides additional useful information. What is more, there is some evidence that certain specific gestures are reliably used to describe a few important symptoms such as a duodenal ulcer's pain, or that from an ischaemic heart (Miller, 1978).

The aspects of non-verbal behaviour which have received most attention in the consultation setting are, however, those concerning the effect of non-verbal behaviour on the interaction of the participants. A complete review of non-verbal behaviour would be inappropriate here, but in considering the role of *touch*, for example, Friedman (1979) summarized in this way:

> . . . touch has various significant functions and meanings in medical settings. Touch may have symbolic value in healing, may create positive expectation, may have important physiological effects, and, even when used for strictly diagnostic purposes, may affect the interpersonal nature of the practitioner-patient interaction. (ibid. p. 89)

The therapeutic effect of touch should not be surprising, moreover, since touch is used by mothers for comfort and guidance and its effects are well documented. *Direction of gaze* serves a number of functions which include both seeking feedback and controlling turns at speaking. Looking can also signify interest or deception and all three roles have significance for consultations. Similarly, *body posture* can communicate interest or concern, and the *seating position* of doctor and patient can significantly influence their communication and the patient's degree of relaxation (Pietroni, 1976). Collectively, the doctor's and patient's non-verbal behaviour significantly determine the impressions each forms of the other. Ben-Sira (1980) investigated the patients' perception of their doctor's feelings and skills in a representative sample of 515 adult urban Israelis. He interviewed them in their homes about a number of issues including their medical care. He found that in patients whose concern about their problem was high, the more similar the doctor's instrumental (skills) and affective behaviour were seen to be. This relationship was weaker in more educated patients but Ben-Sira asserted that a patient's satisfaction with the professional activities of his doctor is determined to a large extent by the doctor's mode of presentation. In short, support from the doctor was a crucial element in patients' evaluation of treatment and its significance increased as the patient's social class decreased.

Friedman *et al.* (1980) studied the non-verbal expressiveness of 21 doctors and found that their expressive ability was significantly correlated with a number of personality traits. Their expressive ability was related to patient satisfaction and the judged likeability of the doctors. Patients were least satisfied with doctors who were perceived as expressing negative emotions when trying to communicate positive ones. Ben-Sira and Friedman *et al.* have, therefore, provided evidence which relates to the role of non-verbal behaviour in medical consultations, but the issue of how accurately the doctor and patient perceive each other's feelings is rarely mentioned.

3.3 The Clinical Process Approach

It is beyond the scope of the present review to detail studies of diagnostic and management decision making or to attempt to resolve the issue of whether a systems approach (Pritchard, 1978) or a pattern recognition approach (Miller, 1978) to clinical problem-solving is the more appropriate. It is appropriate, however, to detail some of the social psychological influences on the clinical process. Stimson (1976) considered some problems for prescribing brought about by the interaction between doctor and patient. He identified four. First, what seems rational to doctor or patient may not seem so to the other. This is a problem for the doctor brought about by the relative lack of feedback between himself and the patient. Secondly, patients' expectations are often not communicated to their doctors for reasons of formality, social distance, lack of time and differences in their language and knowledge. Thirdly, the doctor usually sees the patient away from the social setting of the problem into which the treatment must fit. Finally, the doctor's influence on one patient may be transmitted to others by the patient inappropriately. Melville, we have already seen (1980a,b) demonstrated the influence of the doctor's state on his prescribing but Fielding and Evered (1978) provided evidence that the diagnosis of the same presenting problem may vary according to the perceived socio-economic status of the patient, although their sample of "doctors" was actually of pre-clinical medical students. The diagnosis was more frequently "psychosomatic" with the perceived middle class patient although the study used the "matched guise technique" in which the same person made two audio-tapes and the details of the problem were held constant. The psychological influences on the clinical process, therefore, make diagnosis much less simple than text books of clinical medicine would lead one to believe, and Bennett *et al.* (1979), in their sample of 342 Scottish general practitioners, reported that the majority felt a need for systematized formal training in communication skills.

3.4 The Verbal Content Approach

Argyle *et al.* (1981b) have distinguished between studies of verbal content and studies of utterance types which are content free. The utterance type "questioning", for example, provides no information about the content of the question. In this section, however, verbal descriptive studies of both types will be considered together.

Hays and Larsen (1963) devised a verbal behaviour category scheme for describing the contacts between nurses and patients and Byrne and Long's substantial work on doctor–patient communication was based on Hays and Larson. Byrne and Long (1976; Byrne, 1976; Long, 1974) devised a category scheme for describing the behaviour of doctors rather than patients, in their sample of 2500 audio-taped consultations. Their sample was made up of 60 British G.P.s, five from Holland and six from Ireland. The aim of the research was

> to discover what patterns of behaviour doctors appeared to follow in their consulting rooms and the degree to which the patterns were repetitive among doctors. (Byrne and Long, 1976, p. 21)

They reported that approximately 75% of what took place in their sample was doctor initiated, and that within one continuous hour of any doctor's consultations, he/she would demonstrate 85% of their normal range of behaviours. They drew attention to the discrepancy between what was usually regarded as the standard clinical model of consulting and what was demonstrated in their sample consultations.

The clinical model consisted of achieving rapport, gathering information, forming and validating hypotheses and proposing solutions. What they described was a 6-phase process which consisted of the following: (p. 21)

(1) The doctor establishes a relationship with the patient.

(2) The doctor attempts to discover or actually discovers the reasons for the patient's attendance.

(3) The doctor conducts a verbal or physical examination or both.

(4) The doctor, or the doctor and the patient, or the patient (in order of probability) consider the condition.

(5) The doctor, and occasionally the patient, detail treatment or further investigation.

(6) The consultation is terminated usually by the doctor.

This was the logical sequence of events discovered but some consultations omitted phases, others repeated phases or returned to earlier ones. Five per cent of all consultations appeared not to achieve any discernible objective for either doctor or patient and these were termed dysfunctional consultations. They were characterized by a reduced second phase—a failure accurately to discover the reasons for the patient's attendance. In 8% of consultations the patient introduced another problem when the consultation had apparently ended. This was characterized by an initially reduced phase 2 and then a return to phase 2 when the second problem was introduced. Those doctors who spent

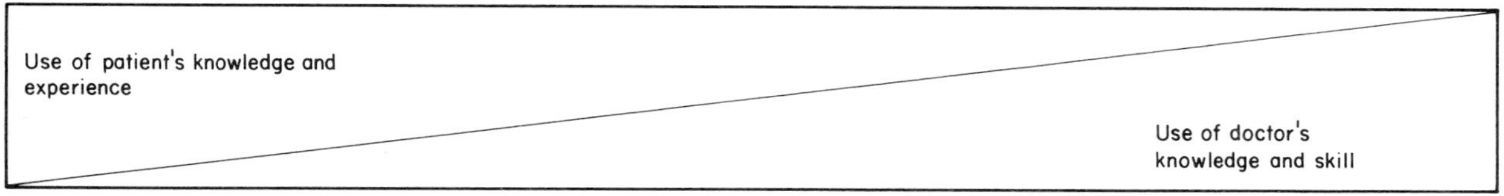

Use of patient's knowledge and experience → **Use of doctor's knowledge and skill**

Silence Listening Reflecting	Clarifying and Interpretation	Analysing and Probing	Gathering information
Offering observation	Broad question	Direct question	Direct question
Encouraging	Clarifying	Correlational question	Closed question
Clarifying	Challenging	Placing events	Correlational question
Reflecting	Repeating for affirmation	Repeating for affirmation	Placing events
Bringing patient ideas	Seeking patient ideas	Suggesting	Summarising to close off
Seeking patient ideas	Offering observation	Offering feeling	Suggesting
Indicating understanding	Concealed question	Exploring	Self-answering questions
Using silence	Placing events	Broad question	Reassuring
	Summarising to open up		Repeating for affirmation
			Justifying self-chastising

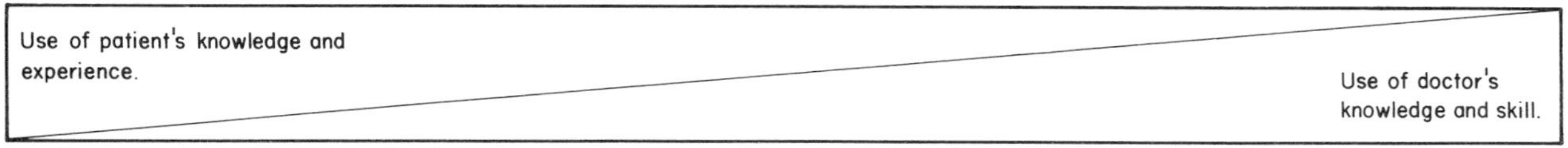

Use of patient's knowledge and experience → **Use of doctor's knowledge and skill**

Doctor permits patients to make decision	Doctor defines the limits and requests the patients to make decision	Doctor presents problem. Seeks suggestions and makes decisions	Doctor presents tentative decision subject to change	Doctor sells his decision to the patient	Doctor makes decision and announces it	Doctor makes decision and instructs patient

Fig. 1.2. Byrne and Long's Diagnostic styles.

relatively more time discovering the reasons for the patient's attendance, got through phases 3, 5 and 6 quicker. There were a number of variables which influenced how long a doctor would spend on phase 2, namely; the prepared-ness of the doctor to accept the first thing the patient said; the degree of clarity of the patient's presentation of symptoms; the number of patients preceding the present one and the number the doctor believed were still to come; the degree to which the doctor was orientated towards organic illness; and the doctor's beliefs about his own and the patient's role. These variables, understandably, include doctor, patient and situation but the consulting style was determined much more by the doctor, that is to say that there were more similarities between the way each doctor dealt with a variety of patients than between types of patient dealt with by a variety of doctors.

Byrne and Long identified styles by clusters of scores in their 55 categories *in specific phases* of the consultation. They described styles, using a power-shift analogy, as ranging from patient centred to doctor centred but they identified four diagnostic styles and seven prescriptive styles along the same continuum. Figure 1.2 describes the diagnostic styles and their characteristic behaviours and identifies the headings of the prescriptive styles.

The relative invariance of style between patients by any doctor suggests a certain rigidity but they maintained that patient centred doctors displayed negative behaviours towards their patients much less frequently than doctor-centred doctors.

One detailed finding reported by Long (1974) to have come out of the work was that, although the mean consultation length was 5·2 min, the distribution was bi-modal with a peak at 3·8 min and a peak at 6·6 min. It is not clear, however, whether this is because of differences between doctors or between serious and non-serious problems.

Bain (1976) audio-taped 480 of his *own* consultations and described their contents. He analysed his verbal behaviour into five categories: social exchange; encouragement; problem resolution; asking questions; giving instructions. The patient's behaviour was analysed into: the presentation of symptoms; answering questions; problem related questions; questions directly about the problem; social exchange. The differences in categories reflect the role difference between doctor and patient. Bain used as his unit of analysis the "unit of expression" so that each detectable separate utterance was scored, like a turn at speaking but any turn may have included more than one unit of expression, such as the answer to a question and a new question. This scoring ignores the length of each utterance. He found that his consultations with patients from social classes 1 and 2 were significantly longer than his consultations with social classes 4 and 5, irrespective of the diagnosis—85 units mean for classes 1 and 2 compared with 52 for 4 and 5. In all consultations, more than 25% consisted of the doctor clarifying the problem or giving instructions and the doctor talked more than the patients. He found differences among consultations dealing with psychiatric problems, chronic conditions and new patients in terms of which behavioural categories were used and to what extent. Later, Bain (1979) analysed the content of 556 consultations from 22 family doctors in the U.S.A. and found that the doctors initiated 80% of the conversation dealing with medical matters and that patients initiated 70% of the conversation which was not strictly medical. Again there was more conversation with upper rather than lower social class patients irrespective of diagnosis. There was also more conversation associated with chronic conditions, emotional disorders and ill-defined conditions.

Stiles *et al.* (1979b) found that it was helpful to divide the consultation into three segments: the medical history, the physical examination and the conclusion. Fifty-two consultations from 19 North American doctors were coded by three coders and eight categories were used: *D*isclosure, *Q*uestion, *E*dification, ac*K*nowledgement, *A*dvisement, *I*nterpretation, *C*onfirmation and *R*eflection. Each utterance was coded for form and intent so that a question which was really intended to provide information for a patient was coded Q(E), for example, "Doesn't your smoking have something to do with your cough?" The researchers compared their categories with a number of other investigations and validity was checked in this way. They found that the doctors talked more than the patients and that there was significant agreement between the coders both for form and intent.

Lucas (1978) investigated specifically the health education information and advice given by 30 British general practitioners in 78 consultations with elderly people. She reported that nearly all consultations contained some health education statement but nearly all of this concerned the presenting problem and its management. Only 2% of statements were directed towards the promotion of health in general, and although 58% of patients were given some advice about their illness, only 15% were given detailed information. Very seldom was any explanation of the reasons for the advice given. In this study, however, differences in the patients' behaviour were ignored although this might have accounted for much of the doctors' behaviour.

3.5 The Evaluative Approach

Evaluation of doctor–patient communication is attempted rarely in the empirical literature but there is a great deal written about what should and should not happen in consultations. The problems are, first, that criteria for evaluation need a clear statement of tasks for the consultation to achieve and this requires evidence of its outcomes. Secondly, any criteria must be well grounded in the empirical literature on the consultation. Finally, the psychometric constraints of reliability and validity should be met by any evaluation scale. This all takes considerable research time and effort. It is relatively easy to offer definitions of what "therapeutic communication" *should* be (e.g. Rossiter, 1975) but quite another thing to satisfy these three requirements.

Raimbault *et al* (1975) reported value loaded findings but this was certainly not an evaluative approach as defined. They analysed just five transcripts of interviews between parents and paediatric endocrinologists. They reported that the doctors and parents were often talking "at cross purposes", that they avoided dealing with the parents' feelings, favouring "quasi-scientific" explanations, and that the doctors were often not aware of the feelings involved, regarding them as beyond their area of competence.

Barsky *et al.* (1980), on the other hand, devised a rating scale of 19 items, which covers the form of the interview, the use of authority, the technique of questioning, the management of the patient's emotions and the information transmitted by the doctor. The values are implicit in the questions and the evaluation by any marking schedule which ignores, as this does, the clinical content of the interview cannot be comprehensive. The questions appear to be repetitive and, in part, irrelevant since the evidence linking the consultation's form to its outcomes is not provided. It only matters that "the doctor moves smoothly between phases of the consultation", for example, if this produces more favourable outcomes such as an increase in patient satisfaction or memory for the doctor's instructions. No psychometric data are available, moreover, so the scale's reliability and validity are open to question. This particular evaluation instrument directs attention, however, to some important aspects of the consultation which are well grounded in the available literature and as psychometric data become available, it may prove to be a useful means of evaluating the non-clinical components of consultations.

3.6 Conclusions and Critique

Process studies provide normative data. This function is valuable and certainly no understanding of any phenomenon is complete without it. The major problems, however, are three-fold. First, there is the problem of which categories should be used. Argyle *et al.* (1981b) have concluded that, while similar categories of social and non-verbal behaviour may well be used in different types of situation, task behaviour is much more situation-specific. Thus, in this case, it may well be important to consider the unique properties of doctor–patient interviews in order to describe their contents appropriately. This is, essentially, the problem of validity. It could be argued, however, that almost any task categories will suffice, so long as they are used by a number of researchers but this does not recognize our repeated argument, that one requirement of process descriptions is that they should be usable in accounting for variance in *outcomes*. If any description cannot account significantly for differences in outcomes from consultations, then its validity must be called into question. Similarly, if any two descriptive schemes account for the same amount of variance in outcomes, they are functionally equivalent. Certainly, sociolinguistic studies are not attempting to account for a consultation's results and if they are to be tested, it may be sufficient to test whether the rules inferred from the observations can be used to generate realistic and legitimate medical conversations. Additionally, the study of non-verbal behaviour in a medical context could be justified as a social psychological investigation in its own right, with little that is unique to the medical setting. If, however, any process descriptive approach is designed to contribute to our specific understanding of medical interviews rather than of language or social interaction in general, then it must be able to show the role of the consultation in its context. To this extent, descriptions of process must be judged against the criterion of accounting for outcomes.

Secondly, descriptions of process must be interpreted in terms of fundamental differences in input such as the nature of the problem. It would be a fruitless exercise to attempt to understand what happened in a series of consultations without considering, in some way, variations in the types of problem which were in hand. Raynes (1980) used the basic distinction between essentially psychological and essentially physical problems to elucidate consultation processes but without this distinction between aspects of input, her study of rituals would have been much less informative.

Thirdly, the analysis of consultation processes is *incomplete*. Process has proved to be an elusive subject of study since sequences are not readily described. Indeed, the promise of a real sequence analysis has yet to be fulfilled. It is possible to describe how much of any particular ingredient is present in a consultation. It is also possible to state where certain ingredients occur but an adequate description of sequences is, at present, beyond the expertise of the behavioural sciences (Argyle *et al.*, 1981a). Markovian analysis allows for the analysis of probabilities that any behavioural event should follow another. It can even extend this estimation of probabilities to three or more steps, but social interaction is almost certainly not organized in strict, left to right sequences. In any statement I make, for example, I can recall an event or a statement which may be two or three sentences back, or even two or three days. In this sense, process descriptions are like the listing of ingredients in a cake without the analysis which shows how to put the ingredients together. For this reason, accounting for variance in a consultation's outcomes may fail either because the categories are unhelpful or because the crucial issue is how the consultation was put together. At present, the best we can do is to describe the ingredients in phases of the consultation—the approach taken by Byrne and Long (1976) and Stiles *et al*. (1979a,b,c). General practice consultations, however, as Byrne and Long discovered, do not fall readily into generalizeable phases as phases may be missing altogether, and Tate (1980) has provided data which suggest that an average of three problems are considered in general practice consultations. For this reason, Stiles' recommendation of a division into history taking, examination and conclusion sections of a consultation is inappropriate to th' study of general practice.

4 OUTCOMES

It has already been noted that outcomes from medical consultations can be immediate, intermediate or long term. This section will confine itself to studies which have measured outcomes with little attempt to relate them to consultation processes.

McGhee (1961) reported that 65% of 400 patients recently discharged from hospital saw communication with medical personnel as the least satisfactory aspect of their hospital stay. In Scott and Gilmore's (1966) study, the main complaint was of a lack of privacy, but neither of these studies attempted seriously to grapple with the need to investigate outcomes systematically and specifically. Satisfaction, for example, is, perhaps, most accurately perceived immediately after any medical contact but it is hard to persuade patients to report dissatisfaction when their need to believe in the treatment is greatest.

4.1 Immediate Out om s

Satisfaction with c᠆᠆ has been extensively studied. A number of recommendations have emerged, therefore, regarding how the measurements should be done. Henley and Davis (1967), for example, suggested a typology for satisfaction measures. Responses to global measures were seen as less sensitive than satisfaction measures for each aspect of an individual's care. There also were composite measures derived from responses to a series of specific items. Usually, scales for measuring satisfaction are composite in nature (Zyzanski *et al*., 1974; Wrigglesworth and Williams, 1975). In Lebow's (1974) review of the literature on patient satisfaction in the United States, it was suggested that, in addition to measuring the patient's subjective perceptions of care, the process, structure, outcomes and impact of care on the patient should also be assessed in order to evaluate the quality of the interaction between doctor and patient. This degree of thoroughness has not usually been followed but

Lebow's contention that it is difficult to get patients to criticize their doctors, is not in dispute. For this reason it is difficult to produce non-reactive satisfaction measures.

Locker and Dunt (1978) have carefully outlined the theoretical and methodological issues in studies of satisfaction with medical care, both in hospital and in general practice. They noticed that patients usually report being satisfied with medical care overall but when asked about specific items, less satisfaction is reported. The communication of information was cited most often as unsatisfactory both in the U.K. and the U.S.A. literature. What is more, the expression of satisfaction was greater in the old than in the young but the relationship with social class was unclear. They did not consider whether there may be an age-by-social-class interaction.

Locker and Dunt (1978) noted that since methods and definitions varied between satisfaction studies it was difficult for comparisons to be made. They recommended that Henley and Davis' typology should be followed and that measurement and analysis should proceed as follows. First, a global measure of satisfaction should be made, followed by free comment on particularly satisfactory and unsatisfactory aspects of care. This will allow the patient's priorities to be noted. Then direct questions should be asked regarding a range of specific aspects of care. An observer should also note any discrepancy between answers to the open and closed questions. The unstructured responses should then be content-analysed into favourable or unfavourable and the ratio calculated. The responses to the closed questions should be in the form of scales. All of these procedures should ensure comparability between types of care and between patients. Finally, a composite measure should be calculated with each of the three components appropriately weighted, but a *post hoc* reduction to a satisfied/dissatisfied dichotomy should be avoided since it is insensitive. When evaluations are made, therefore, the full range of satisfaction should be evaluated rather than concentrating on either the very dissatisfied or the very satisfied (Shaw, 1976). In the case of general practice, they concluded, satisfaction was most appropriately measured immediately after specific consultations rather than attempting to measure general satisfaction with medical care (e.g. Hulka *et al.*, 1971).

Their theoretical considerations were equally helpful. Satisfaction is rarely defined. Stimson and Webb (1975) suggested that satisfaction was related to the patient's perception of the outcome of treatment and the extent to which the treatment met the patient's expectations. There was much evidence, however, that the patient's expectations and satisfaction had more to do with the process of care and the personal qualities of the doctor rather than the consultation's clinical content.

This contention certainly is implicit in Wolf *et al.* (1978) who report the development of a U.S.A. medical interview satisfaction scale consisting of 26 items which cover the cognitive (information), affective (feelings/empathy) and behavioural aspects of a consultation.

The other extensively investigated immediate outcome of care is the patient's memory of the doctor's instructions. Reynolds (1978) is typical of many investigators in reporting a large number of patients who would like more information, and lack of information was said to lead to anxiety and fear. The literature has tended to concentrate, however, on the extent of patients' recall of what the doctor *did* tell them, despite reports such as that of Woods (1979). Woods questioned 100 patients about to undergo surgery to discover the patients' knowledge of procedures they were about to undergo and what they would be expected to do before, during and after admission to hospital. He took, as a criterion of preparedness, the patients' ability to answer correctly a set of 12 questions and discovered that only one patient was fully informed.

Factors associated with recall of the doctors instructions and information have included aspects of the consultation (see below), the patient, the problem and the therapy. Brody (1980) for example, found that *low* recall of the therapeutic regimen was associated with relatively *greater* discomfort and *lower* activity level in the patient, *more* prescribed medications and ancillary measures and *less* satisfaction with the doctor.

Ley (Chapter 4, this volume) has reviewed his own and others' research on the matter of patients' recall. This work clearly supports the finding of several studies that patients are dissatisfied with the information they receive, even when doctors make (untrained) efforts to improve the situation (Hugh-Jones *et al.*, 1964; Spelman *et al.*, 1966; Houghton, 1968). Forgetting was associated with the amount of information presented, the nature of the material, the patient's age, level of anxiety and level of medical knowledge. Evidence relating memory to the consultation will be presented below.

4.2 Intermediate Outcomes

The major intermediate outcome, which has received extensive attention has been compliance with the doctor's instructions (Cohen, 1979). Assessment of patient compliance is carried out in a number of ways: biological measures, subjective ratings, self-report, pill counts and direct observation (Dunbar, 1979). Since no method is optimal, Dunbar recommends the use of multiple measures for more complete data. She also categorizes the three basic approaches to defining compliance. The first is a quantitative assessment of the degree to which a regimen was followed—usually expressed as a ratio or percentage. Hulka, for example, has identified four types of medication errors: missing out pills which should be taken, taking extra pills, misunderstanding the schedule and ignoring the schedule (Hulka *et al.*, 1975; Hulka *et al.*, 1976).

The second approach is categorical where patients are said to be good, poor or non-compliers and should be based upon an objective measure rather than subjective impressions. The third is to establish a composite index of compliance based on behaviour, knowledge and possibly even the attitudes of the complier. Unfortunately, the literature on compliance has not identified any *one* method as being preferable which makes comparison difficult. Ley (Chapter 4, this volume) has indicated the extent of the non-compliance problem in a summary of three comprehensive reviews. Similar findings are reported for antenatal and dietary advice (Ley, 1972).

The reasons why patients do not comply have been investigated both by searching for correlations and by experimentation. The Carnegie Grant Sub-committee on the Modification of Patient Behaviour for Health Maintenance and Disease Control (Becker *et al.*, 1977) thoroughly reviewed the relevant literature and compared eight models which could potentially be used to explain "health actions". They chose the Health Belief Model (see Chapter 5 by King, this volume) for several reasons. First, it suggested modifiable links between demographic variables and the utilization of health care services. Secondly, it was soundly based theoretically, essentially on the psychology of motivation (Lewin *et al.*, 1944). Thirdly, it focussed on the perceived valence of health goals and the subjective probability of attainment. Fourthly, it could be used to explain preventive health actions as well as illness and sick-role behaviour. Finally, there were aspects of the HBM in the other models the committee considered. Certainly the HBM variables have been used successfully to predict compliance. Becker (1979) reviewed 30 studies which had investigated the efficacy of HBM variables in accounting for variance in compliance and reported that in 29 of the studies one or more HBM variable was significantly associated with the dependent measure. The review considered studies of the relationship between patients' knowledge, their demographic circumstances, and their attitudes on compliance and concluded that the HBM was the best predictor.

4.3 Long-term Outcomes

Improvement in the patient's health, we have already seen, may be an unhelpful notion in the context of general practice (see Section 1 above). Britton *et al.* (1980) investigated benefits from medical intervention in a Swedish outpatient clinic. Seventy-six patients were followed-up twelve months after treatment. Care was said to be successful only when it made them feel better or improved their prognosis. This occurred in two-out-of-three patients. The rest improved spontaneously, remained unchanged or deteriorated. The authors recommended that patient satisfaction was important in evaluating care but that, "to justify medical care, . . . improvement in the patient's health or prognosis must also be obtained" (p. 484).

Long-term clinical outcomes would be inappropriate to consider here in detail. Irvine *et al*. (1980) have reviewed the available literature. Other long-term outcomes, we shall see, are difficult to relate to process with the exception of changes in the patient's health understanding.

5 PROCESSES AND OUTCOMES

Donabedian (1967) considered the role of outcome as an indicator of quality of care. The problems of using outcome to serve this evaluative purpose were, first, that any particular outcome may not be appropriate for all conditions. An example would be that survival is not an appropriate outcome measure in non life-threatening conditions. Secondly, medical care is limited in its function. A long period of time may have to elapse before an outcome is manifest and other factors may have an influence during this time. Thirdly, some outcomes are hard to measure. Amongst these, Donabedian included patients' attitudes and satisfaction, social restoration of function and rehabilitation. Finally, variations in outcome do not give insight into those specific deficiencies or strengths to which the outcome may be attributed. Despite these problems, Donabedian maintained: "Outcomes, by and large, remain the ultimate validators of the effectiveness and quality of medical care" (p. 169).

Donabedian also considered the role of the administrative structure in which care is provided and the care process. He concluded that:

> . . . before one can make judgements about quality, one needs to understand how patients and physicians interact and how physicians function in the process of providing care. Once the elements of process and their interrelationships are understood, one can attach value judgements to them in terms of their contributions to intermediate and ultimate goals. (p. 193).

Donabedian's more recent work has maintained most of these basic distinctions (Donabedian, 1980).

Clinical outcomes have been reviewed by Irvine *et al*. (1980) and are beyond the scope of this present review. This section will consider the role of process in determining immediate outcomes (5.1), intermediate outcomes (5.2) and longer term outcomes (5.3).

5.1 Process and Immediate Outcomes

A study conducted in California, attempted to relate patient satisfaction and compliance to aspects of process (Freemon *et al.*, 1971; Korsch *et al.*, 1971; Korsch and Negrete, 1972). A total of over 800 paediatric interviews were audio-taped and the mothers were interviewed after their consultations. The audio-tapes were then analysed according to the category system devised by Bales (1950), which divides the behaviour of doctor and patient into 12 discrete categories which cover their socio-emotional and task behaviour. Satisfaction was then related to the incidence of doctors' and patients' behaviour in the 12 categories (the results are summarized in Table 1.1) Korsch and colleagues (1968) had already demonstrated that only 36% of those who received no reassurance during the consultation were satisfied, and Korsch and Negrete (1972) reported that the most frequent statement of dissatisfaction was that the doctor showed too little interest in their concern about their child. Indeed, 26% of the mothers stated that they had not voiced their greatest concern to their doctor at all because they did not have an opportunity or were not encouraged to do so, although only 54 mothers out of the 800 interviewed questioned the doctors' technical competence. A specific finding of particular interest was that a lot of warmth rather than the maintenance of authority on the doctor's part was associated with satisfaction and compliance. Satisfaction was not related to the length of the consultation, but was related to its content.

Kupst *et al.* (1975) found no consultation correlates of patient satisfaction or on anxiety reduction but this finding was unusual. Larsen and Rootman (1976) found support for a hypothesis derived from role theory which suggested that satisfaction with medical care would be influenced by the degree to which a doctor's behaviour corresponded with the patient's expectations of his role. In this study by questionnaire of 757 respondents, the predicted relationship was demonstrated even when demographic variables and frequency of contact were held constant.

Van Dorp (1977) reported an extensive project in Holland to define the skills of interviewing patients, devise ways of measuring them, and then train medical students to use them. He defined behavioural category types of the doctor's behaviour and then used factor analysis to reduce the data to three factors which explained a third of the *total* variance. The first factor he called directed and factual questioning; the second, sympathetic and encouraging questioning, and the third, domination. He then interviewed the patients and had the consultations rated by independent judges. When the behavioural scores were added to the interview and rating data, that is, combining measures which were to be treated as independent with dependent measures, four dimensions were produced by a further factor analysis. These Van Dorp indentified as:

(1) satisfaction and confidence on the patient's part;
(2) the "tempo" of the discussion;
(3) domination on the part of the interviewer;

(4) clarity of questions.

From these analyses, demonstrably reliable and valid evaluation measures were derived. He found that directive techniques used by the medical students provided more information but were negatively associated with the satisfaction of the patient and were not associated with better case presentations—that is, they did not provide further insight into the patients' problems. Empathic techniques, by contrast, were related to the satisfaction of the patient.

Woolley *et al.* (1978) studied the relationships between the patients' expectations, doctor–patient communication about expectations, patient satisfaction, compliance and functional outcomes of care. The sample was of 1761 acute primary care consultations. The patients were interviewed both before and after their consultations, and a follow-up interview was also conducted at a date determined by the doctor's estimate of when benefits of his action would occur. The doctors were only interviewed after the consultation and the consultation was not recorded. Overall, Woolley *et al.* report "few meaningful correlations". The findings, reported in Table 1.1, were from discriminant analysis. It should be mentioned, however, that only 4% of the patients were not satisfied with care and this would make the discriminant analysis less than optimal. They concluded that the degree to which the patient feels the doctor cares about him may well be the most important element in determining satisfaction and compliance.

Stiles *et al.* (1979a, 1979c) and Wolf *et al.* (1978) distinguished between cognitive (information), affective (feelings) and behavioural satisfaction. "Behavioural satisfaction" has to do with the conduct of a physical examination as well as the overall pace of the interview. They report finding, in 52 initial consultations, that affective satisfaction was associated with the free transmission of information from patient to doctor early on in the consultation. Cognitive satisfaction, on the other hand, was associated with the transmission of information about the illness and treatment from doctor to patient in the latter part of the consultation. They used factor analysis of the doctors' and of the patients' behaviour in the consultation and then correlated each factor with the satisfaction outcome measures.

DiMatteo *et al.* (1979) asked 342 patients to rate the doctors they had just seen on nine performance-variables which included the doctor's manner, and intelligence as well as the types of questions asked and how much care the doctor displayed. They also asked the patients whether they intended to see the same doctor again. They found that patients were more likely to want to return to see a doctor who was rated high on socio-emotional (feeling) variables and that there was no effect of the ratings of the doctor's intelligence. What is more, there was a lower correlation between decision to return and the ratings of the doctor's listening and explanations in patients with more serious problems. Other findings are summarized in Table 1.1. Similarly, Ben-Sira

(1980) interviewed 515 Israelis to determine their reactions to recent medical care. The questions asked covered the physician's skills, behaviour and emotional involvement. He found that patients who were more worried about their illness distinguished less between satisfaction with the doctor's skills and with his "affective behaviour" (feelings). This was also true of less educated patients.

Friedman *et al.* (1980) reported finding that a doctor's general ability to express emotions non-verbally was significantly correlated with a number of personality traits. They then went on to investigate the relationships between patient satisfaction and the doctor's expressive ability, and found the expected positive relationship. They demonstrated, moreover, that patients were less satisfied with those doctors who had been perceived to be expressing negative emotions when trying to communicate positive ones. This finding does not, however, lead to the conclusion that, since personality is relatively stable over time, nothing can be done to improve the expressive ability of the doctors involved. Evidence from the literature on psychotherapy has demonstrated how the attributes of the effective psychotherapist can be successfully learned through training (Truax and Carkhuff, 1967; Truax and Mitchell, 1971).

Ley (see Chapter 4 this volume) has reviewed a number of studies which have demonstrated that satisfaction with communication is associated with the patients' understanding of the instructions given. This paper is primarily concerned with understanding and recall of medical information. Ley presents considerable evidence to show that recall is aided by dividing the information into clear categories, and by repetition of the information. Ley demonstrates that specific advice is recalled more accurately than general advice and that combinations of all three of these techniques produce significant improvements in communication effectiveness. Hulka *et al.* (1975) have reported that memory of instructions about the management of diabetes is associated with the method of treatment and how long the patient has had the problem. This is probably due to the specificity and importance of the advice as well as the number of times the information has been given. It is uncommon, however, for one type of problem alone to be used in research of this kind.

Bertakis (1977) has provided corroborative evidence that recall and satisfaction with communication are both increased when patients are asked to repeat instructions given and the doctor gives feedback. Liptack *et al.* (1977) provided additional evidence that satisfaction with care is associated with recall of information. Bain (1977), by contrast, showed that patients from higher social classes recall information better than patients from lower social classes. Anderson (1979), however, investigated recall of information in 151 rheumatology out-patients. He reported that more information was recalled about treatment than about diagnosis and that the overall proportion recalled was 40%. What is more, the doctors estimated correctly that the patients forgot

Table 1.1. Studies relating patient satisfaction to process.

Study	Aspect of satisfaction	Variables shown to be related
Korsch et al. (1968)	dissatisfaction	no reassurance
Freemon et al. (1971)	satisfaction	proportion of Dr talk high Dr behaviour warm and friendly Dr volunteered information Dr discussed causes of problem patient expressed agreement and understanding much social chat
Korsch et al. (1971) Korsch and Negrete (1972)	satisfaction	Dr showed friendly interest Dr discovered concerns Dr dealt with expectations Dr gave specific instructions Dr offered continued support Dr expressed trust in caretaking ability of mother
Kupst et al. (1975)	satisfaction	none
Larsen and Rootman (1976)	satisfaction	Dr conformed to patients' expectations
Roter (1977)	dissatisfaction	increased patient questioning after experimental intervention
Van Dorp (1977)	dissatisfaction	Dr asked many closed questions
	satisfaction	Dr used empathic questions
Woolley et al. (1978)	satisfaction with care	satisfaction with outcome continuity of care communication about patient expectations patient expectations fulfilled
	satisfaction with outcome	actual outcome satisfaction with care
Romm and Hulka (1979)	satisfaction	patient memory of specific information
Stiles et al. (1979)	"affective" satisfaction	patient explained condition in own words early in interview
	"cognitive" satisfaction	Dr freely informed patient about illness and treatment at end of interview

Study	Aspect of satisfaction	Variables shown to be related
Di Matteo *et al.* (1979)	patient's positive evaluation of doctors' behaviour	patients' age patients' sex patients' occupational status patients' level of education
	patients' expressed willingness to return to same doctor	patients' positive evaluation of doctor's behaviour seriousness of problem
Ben-Sira (1980)	patients' positive evaluation of doctor's behaviour	patients' degree of concern about problem patients' level of education
Friedman *et al.* (1980)	satisfaction	aspects of doctor's personality doctor's non-verbal expressiveness
Ley (Chapter 4, this volume)	satisfaction with communication	understanding of instructions

most of what they were told. There was no difference between men and women in the proportion of information recalled. Increasing age was not associated with forgetting except in the over 70s, and working-class and middle-class patients remembered the same proportion of information given. The only aspect of the illness to be associated with better recall was in the recall of aspects of the treatment. This was higher in the group who had experienced more severe pain. Patients who rated themselves as more anxious during the consultation recalled significantly more. Anderson then categorized each of a group of 29 of the consultations into one of four categories based on how much the patient participated in the consultation. The categories varied from "monologue" in which the doctor was active and the patient passive, to "dialogue" in which the doctor and the patient were both active. No significant relationship was demonstrated, however, between these categories and the amount remembered.

In summary, it would seem that satisfaction of the patient is more likely when the doctor discovers and deals with the patient's concerns and expectations; when the doctors' manner communicates warmth, interest and concern about the patient; when the doctor volunteers a lot of information and explains things to the patient in terms that are understood. Similarly, patients are more likely to recall medical information when it is presented simply, specifically, in explicit categories, and when it is repeated.

5.2 Process and Intermediate Outcomes

The emphasis in the literature on the study of compliance as an intermediate outcome is interesting in as much as it seems based on the assumption that compliance is to be encouraged. This may be so but the case should be made rather than merely assumed to be true. Should it be that compliance is not associated with the benefit of reduced morbidity or improvement in condition, compliance would be, at best, unimportant and, at worst, undesirable. This is a matter for medical scientists to discover in the evaluation of therapeutic regimes. An additional measure they might consider, however, is whether or not compliance may be gained at the expense of self-reliance on the patient's part. If this were to be the case, the increasing of patient compliance would be tantamount to the encouragement of doctor dependence. Further consideration of this matter, however, would be inappropriate here.

Davis (1966) investigated the congruence between doctors' estimates of their patients' compliance and patients' compliance reported in empirical studies. In his sample of 131 physicians, 42% of them believed that almost all of their patients complied and that there was not much difference in compliance rates among different types of patient. The empirical studies had demonstrated, however, that 35% of patients were to be classed as non-compliers. What is more, the doctors attributed non-compliance to the patients: either *they* were unable to understand or *they* were uncooperative. More recent evidence on the extent of the non-compliance of patients has been presented by Ley (see Chapter 4, this volume) who has demonstrated that there is a large range of non-compliance with many forms of medication and treatment and that usually half of the doctor's instructions are not carried out.

Davis (1968) investigated the relationship between compliance and the content of the consultation. Certain evidence was cited that some patient characteristics affected compliance: for example, women defaulted more, as did older people and people from lower socio-economic groups. Patients with urgent acute illnesses and patients with long-term illnesses, who had received careful instruction, by contrast, complied more. Davis also provided evidence that aspects of the therapeutic regime and the influence of other people affected compliance. He carried out the study in question, however, since it was his expressed view that the evidence, regarding the role of doctor–patient communication in producing compliance, was inconclusive. The study consisted of 154 new patients and the same number of doctors. Four different types of measure were used:

(1) Part of each patient's consultation and the whole of their revisits were

audio-taped and the tapes were analysed. The proportion of talk by doctor and patient was ascertained and the tapes were coded to discover how much of each of Bales' (1950) behavioural types were apparent. By manipulating category scores, indexes of communication difficulty in each consultation were derived. Finally, the behavioural coding was subjected to a factor analysis to reveal the underlying dimensions.

(2) Personal interviews with patients and self-administered questionnaires with the doctors were carried out before and after the first consultations and after the second and third consultations.

(3) Six months later, the patients' medical records were used to obtain information about the type of regimen recommended, the number of broken appointments, and the patients' demographic circumstances.

(4) A composite index of compliance was calculated so as to allow for the weighted importance of each aspect of the regime and the patients' degree of compliance with it.

The results demonstrated that 37% of the patients were non-compliant and that none of the demographic characteristics measured was significantly associated with compliance. The factor analysis produced ten factors from the doctors' and patients' behaviour combined. There was no significant relationship between behaviour in the initial consultation and the future compliance of the patients—possibly because not all of the consultation was available for analysis. Compliance was significantly correlated, however, with five of the ten factors of behaviour in the re-visits. The first significant factor was called "malintegrative behaviour" and was characterized by over-formality and general negative emotions. The second significant factor was called "active patient-permissive doctor" and represented interaction between an authoritarian patient and a doctor who passively accepted this situation. The third factor demonstrated to be significant was called "nondirective antagonism" and was typified by the doctor who showed some antagonism to the patient and who neglected to give the patient information and explanations, confining his activity to expressing opinions. Significant factor four was named "non-reciprocal informativeness" and reflected the doctor who gathered much information from the patient while the patient co-operated in this but the doctor did not reciprocate by giving information and explanations to the patient. These four factors were significantly correlated with *non*-compliance. The factor which was significantly correlated with compliance was called "tension release" but was really a more positive combination of behaviours than the name implies in which the doctor and patient joked with each other, laughed, and demonstrated some satisfaction with the relationship.

Davis' study was the first of its kind to use factors in trying to predict compliance. This approach makes good use of the data but at the time, multivariate techniques, such as multiple regression, were not widely in use.

Multiple regression would certainly have helped to clarify the picture since it would have determined how much compliance could be predicted from combinations of the factors. At the moment we do not know the extent to which each factor contributes uniquely to the prediction of compliance. Korsch and her colleagues (Korsch and Negrete, 1972; Korsch *et al.*, 1971; Freemon *et al.*, 1971; Francis *et al.*, 1969), in the studies reported earlier concerning satisfaction and compliance, found that compliance was predicted well by the patients' satisfaction. Compliance was also related to doctors who explained things to the mothers and who fulfilled the mothers' expectations. Non-compliance was associated with the doctors' failure to show friendly interest.

The relationship between satisfaction and compliance was also demonstrated in the U.K. by Kincey *et al.* (1975) who additionally demonstrated that compliance was related to the patients' understanding of the doctors' instructions. This finding was replicated by Ley *et al.* (1976) and Ley (1980). Clearly, patients cannot comply with information they do not remember or do not understand.

On this theme, medication errors have been related to misunderstanding and poor memory of specific instructions, as well as to the number of drugs prescribed and the complexity of the schedule (Hulka *et al.*, 1975, 1976). No effect of patient characteristics on compliance was discovered, moreover, leading to the conclusion that effective communication of information and instructions was the major contributor to the taking of the medication appropriately. Romm and Hulka (1979), however, took a rather more ambitious approach to the data. Using the data from the earlier studies, they investigated the relationship between process and outcome of care, this time making use of multivariate statistics. The measures they identified as process measures were:

(1) The doctor's awareness of the patient's concerns, expressed as a ratio after interviewing each party.

(2) The information remembered by the patient, expressed as a percentage of what the doctor said he had told the patient. This was called "communication".

(3) The drug error rate of each patient.

(4) The doctor's adherence to minimum care criteria. This was made possible since only diabetes management was under investigation.

(5) The extent to which the patients utilized the care services.

Some of these measures, however, notably 2, 3 and 5, are more strictly to be seen as outcome measures. The investigators' use of the term outcomes was confined in this study to the level of diabetic control and the patients' overall satisfaction with the doctor and the care received. They report several significant, but small, correlations between a number of their measures but, when multiple regression was used, it revealed little that was significant and it accounted for very little variance in the outcome measures. This finding led the authors to conclude that the process measures used in the study were inadequate predictors of patient outcomes. Earlier, however, Romm *et al.* (1976) had demonstrated that, in a sample of patients with congestive heart failure, process measures had significantly predicted outcomes in those patients who were less ill than the average.

Roter (1977) *manipulated* the amount patients asked and received answers to their questions in consultations. She trained patients, immediately before they saw the doctor, to formulate concisely their concerns and ideas about the information they wanted, into questions. This raised significantly the amount of questions the patients asked in their consultations compared with a control group. What is more, the experimental group showed a significantly higher appointment keeping (compliance) ratio than the control group, but the experimental group's consultations were characterized by the increased display of negative feelings, specifically anxiety and anger, compared with the control group's consultations, which were characterized as mutually sympathetic. The experimental group, moreover, expressed less satisfaction with care despite their higher compliance rate. This North American study seemed to show that satisfaction is not a necessary precondition of compliance. What is unclear is whether the questions generated the negative feelings or whether they were a product of a disruption of the normal pattern of consultations. Certainly, it should be remembered that Francis *et al.* (1969) had demonstrated that compliance and satisfaction were related to the volunteering of explanations by the doctor. More research would therefore appear to be needed to determine the conditions under which doctors volunteer information to patients. This question was investigated extensively by Waitzkin and Stoeckle (1972, 1976).

Ley (1976) had maintained that there was considerable dispute about how effective it was to arouse fear in patients to increase compliance. Kirscht *et al.* (1978), however, investigated the effects of the degree of "threat" or fear arousal in the information the doctor gave and of the mothers' health beliefs on producing weight loss in obese children. The dependent measure was, arguably, a guide to the mothers' compliance. The mothers were all from low income homes. The authors reported that the high threat messages did, in fact, produce the most consistent weight loss. They also reported that the children lost most weight whose mothers' health beliefs were salient to the subject of obesity. They conjectured that good doctor–patient communication had served to make the beliefs salient and, therefore, increase the probability of action. The mothers' beliefs about the value of medical care was related to appointment keeping. Hutchinson (1979), on the other hand, had demonstrated that patients who are involved in measuring their *own* blood pressure, and who detect that it is raised, consult their doctors about it quite reliably.

David Pendleton

This, rather unusually, could be seen as an example of compliance with the result of the patients' own diagnostic evaluation.

In summary: there is evidence relating compliance to a number of variables. The patients' expectations and beliefs, the complexity of the treatment plan,

Table 1.2. Studies relating patient compliance to process.

Study	Aspect of compliance	Variables shown to be related
Davis (1968)	non-compliance	doctors's and patient's behaviour not well integrated in re-visit: active patient-permissive doctor non-directive antagonism non-reciprocal informativeness
	compliance	tension release
Francis et al. (1969)	compliance	patients' expectations fulfilled physicians' explanations
Freemon et al. (1971)	compliance	patients' satisfaction
Korsch et al. (1971)		patients' expectations fulfilled
	non-compliance	doctor fails to show friendly interest
Kincey et al. (1975)	compliance	comprehension of doctor's instructions patients' satisfaction
Hulka et al. (1975) (1976)	medication errors	number of drugs prescribed complexity of schedule patients' lack of knowledge of drug function
Hulka, Kupper et al. (1975)	kept appointments and medication errors in diabetics	memory for certain specific instructions re diabetes
Ley et al. (1976)	compliance	patients' satisfaction comprehension of doctor's instructions
Roter (1977)	compliance	amount patient questions doctor
Kirscht et al. (1978)	weight loss in children	amount of threat in message to mother mother's health beliefs
	appointment keeping	belief in value of medical care
Wolf et al. (1978)	compliance	patients' satisfaction
Ley (1980)	compliance	comprehension of doctor's instructions

the patients' understanding and memory of the doctors' instructions and the patients' overall degree of satisfaction all play their part. Aspects of the consultation are clearly related to compliance but, as yet, we do not know whether these influence compliance directly or through the immediate outcomes they produce. The model proposed in Fig. 1.1 would suggest that compliance will be determined by those immediate outcomes which collectively would be said to constitute the patients psychological reaction to the consultation. Table 1.2 summarizes the major studies relating the consultation to patient compliance.

Other studies relating consultation processes to intermediate outcomes are those of Janis (1958) and Egbert *et al.* (1964) who showed that, when patients are given information before an operation concerning what to expect after the operation is over, they require fewer analgesics and report less pain. Similarly, Liptack *et al.* (1977) showed that patients' adaptation to their problems was positively correlated with the doctor's awareness of their concerns. The evidence, therefore, suggests that coping is made easier when the patient feels understood and is well informed. Miller (1980), however, has presented evidence that there may be a fundamental difference between people who cope best when they are told what to expect as against those who seek to distract themselves from warning signals.

5.3 Process and Long-term Outcomes

It is not surprising that patients whose condition improves express satisfaction with the outcome and the care they have received (Woolley *et al.*, 1978). When patients ultimately decide to change their doctors, however, Mechanic (1964) reported that they more frequently complained of the doctor's lack of interest, care and motivation than of his medical acumen. Romm *et al.* (1976), moreover, had demonstrated a relationship between improvement in the patients' condition and the doctors' awareness of the patients' problems. For a review of longer-term clinical outcomes see Irvine *et al.* (1980).

6 CONCLUSIONS

It was argued at the beginning of this chapter that research into complex phenomena, such as doctor–patient communication, is inevitably fragmented. No individual study could hope to do justice to all of the complexities and yet the absence of an adequate theory or model has made it difficult to build up a composite understanding from the studies of its parts.

The chapter has presented the findings of a considerable number of investigations into various aspects of the consultation. The review of the literature has also revealed several important problems. First, there is the need to know how best to interrelate the studies. Integration, we have argued, will require a MODEL, however simple, which can be used both to organize the literature which is already available and to suggest directions for future research. The simple input–process–outcome model which has been proposed (Fig. 1.1) has been used to organize the literature in this chapter and the exercise has revealed a number of important omissions, such as research on the way the doctor perceives the consultation and its outcomes. The model goes further, however, since it suggests a *sequence of effects*. The model suggests that input variables will affect the consultation processes, that the doctor and the patient will influence each other and that the process will affect the consultation's outcomes. Similarly, the model suggests that immediate outcomes will affect later outcomes but predicts that the effect will become weaker as the time increases between the consultation and the outcome in question. This is important since, for example, McAuliffe (1978) has recently felt the need to defend the link between process and outcome in the light of studies which have failed to find such correlations. Romm and Hulka (1979), moreover, have implied that process and outcome measures may have to be considered as independent. In direct contrast, the model would suggest that the consultation will have clear effects, the clearest of which will be found in its *immediate outcomes*, since more distant outcomes are subject to other powerful effects.

Secondly, the literature review has failed to find an adequate formulation of consultation processes in terms of SOCIAL INTERACTION. Such a formulation would be psychological in its content, rather than, for example, socio-demographic or socio-linguistic. It would also be dynamic in nature, that is, it would describe the processes at work rather than the more fixed entities such as social status or health beliefs. Much of the research on health beliefs, it will be remembered, has simply looked for the effect of the patient's health beliefs on what the patient does, rather than go on to address itself to the reciprocal effect of the subsequent behaviour, or the behaviour of others, on the patient's health beliefs. A formulation of consultation processes in terms of social interaction would clarify the role of the consultation as a transaction or mutual social influence process and would lead to an expectation that the consultation would bring about changes in the participants. Such changes might be expected in their knowledge, their moods and their subsequent behaviour.

Thirdly, any adequate formulation should be PRACTICAL. The consultation entails a working relationship and to understand its processes would be to entertain the possibility of improving its effectiveness. Thus, training in consultation skills should derive from the model and the research it spawns.

REFERENCES

Anderson, J. L. (1979). Patients' recall of information and its relation to the nature of the consultation. In *Research in Psychology and Medicine* (Oborne *et al.*, eds). Academic Press, London.

Argyle, J. M. (1969). *Social Interaction*. Methuen, London.

Argyle, J. M. (1975). *Bodily Communication*. International Universities Press, New York.

Argyle, J. M. Clark, D. D. and Collett, P. (1981a). The *Sequential Analysis of Social Behaviour Applied to Social Skills and Group Conflict*. Final report to the Social Science Research Council, London, S.S.R.C.

Argyle, J. M., Furnham, A. F. and Graham, J. G. (1981b). *Social Situations*. Cambridge University Press, Cambridge.

Bain, D. J. (1976). Doctor–patient communication in general practice consultations. *Med. Ed.* **10** (2), 125–131.

Bain, D. J. (1977). Patient knowledge and the content of the consultation in general practice. *Med. Ed.* **11** (5), 347–350.

Bain, D. J. (1979). The content of physician-patient communication in family practice. *J. Fam. Pract.* **8** (4), 745–753.

Bales, R. F. (1950). *Interaction Process Analysis: A Method for the Study of Small Groups*. Addison-Wesley, Cambridge, Mass.

Balint, M. (1964). *The Doctor, his Patient and the Illness*. Pitman, London.

Barsky, A. J., Kazis, L. E., Freiden, R. B., Goroll, A. H., Hatem, C. J. and Lawrence, R. S. (1980). Evaluating the interview in primary care medicine. *Soc. Sci. Med.* **14A**, 653–658.

Becker, M. H. (1979). Understanding patient compliance: the contributions of attitudes and other psychosocial factors. In *New Directions in Patient Compliance* (S. Cohen, ed.). Lexington Books, U.S.A.

Becker, M. H., Haefner, D. P., Kasl, S. V., Kirscht, J. P., Maiman, L. A. and Rosenstock, I. M. (1977). Selected psychosocial models and correlates of individual health-related behaviours. *Med. Care* **15** (5), supp. 27–46.

Bennett, A., Knox, J. D. E. and Morrison, A. T. (1978). Difficulties in consultations reported by doctors in general practice. *J. Roy. Coll. Gen. Prac.* **28**, 646–651.

Bennett, A., Morrison, A. J. and Knox, J. D. (1979). Common sense and consulting. *J. Roy. Coll. Gen. Prac.* **29** (201), 209–215.

Ben-Sira, Z. (1980). Affective and instrumental components in the physician-patient relationship. *J. Health Soc. Behav.* **21**, 170–180.

Bertakis, K. D. (1977). The communication of information from physician to patient: a method for increasing patient retention and satisfaction. *J. Fam. Prac.* **5** (2), 217–222.

Birdwhistell, R. L. (1952). *Introduction to Kinesics*. University of Louisville Press, Louisville.

Boer, R. A. de (1973). *Nascholing van Huisartsen*. Boom.

Boranic, M. (1979). Silent information. *J. Med. Ethic.* **5** (2), 80–82.

Boreham, P. and Gibson, D. (1978). The informative process in private medical consultations: a preliminary investigation. *Soc. Sci. Med.* **12** (5A), 409–416.

Britton, M., Orth-Gomer, K. and Rehnqvist, N. (1980). Patient benefits from medical measures: results in an outpatient clinic for internal medicine. *Soc. Sci. Med.* **14A**, 481–484.

Brody, D. (1980). An analysis of patient recall of their therapeutic regimens. *J. Chronic Dis.* **33**, 57–63.

Browne, R. B. (1978). Patient and professional interaction and its relationship to patients' health status and frequent use of health services. *Diss. Abstr. Inter.* **39** (4A), 2075.

Bruhn, J. A. and Trevino, F. M. (1979). A method for determining patients' perceptions of their health needs. *J. Fam. Prac.* **8**, 809–818.

Byrne, P. (1976). Teaching and learning verbal behaviours. In: *Language and communication in general practice*, Tanner, B. (Ed.) pp. 52–70. London: Hodder and Stoughton.

Byrne, P. S. and Long, B. E. L. (1976). *Doctors Talking to Patients.* H.M.S.O., London.

Cartwright, A. (1964). *Human Relations and Hospital Care.* Routledge and Kegan Paul, London.

Cartwright, A. and Anderson, R. (1979). *Patients and their Doctors in 1977. J. Roy. Coll. Gen. Prac.*, London.

Cartwright, A. and Anderson, R. (1981). *General Practice Revisited.* Tavistock Publications, London.

Cartwright, A. and O'Brien, M. (1976). Social class variations in health care and in the nature of general practitioner consultations. In *The Sociology of the N.H.S. Sociological Review Monograph* (M. Stacey, ed.). No. 22, University of Keele.

Cassell, E. J., Skopek, L. and Fraser, B. (1977). A preliminary model for the examination of doctor–patient communication. *Language Sci.* **43**, 10–13.

Coe, R. M. (1970). *Sociology of Medicine.* McGraw-Hill, New York.

Cohen, S. (ed.). (1979). *New Directions in Patient Compliance.* Lexington Books, New York.

Collett, P. (ed.) (1979). *Social Rules and Social Behaviour.* Blackwell, Oxford.

Coope, J. and Metcalfe, D. (1979). How much do patients know? A MCQ paper for patients in the waiting room. *J. Roy. Coll. Gen. Prac.* **29** (205), 482–488.

Coulthard, M. and Ashby, M. (1975). Talking with the doctor, 1. *J. Commun.* **25** (3), 140–147.

Crystal, D. (1976). The diagnosis of sociolinguistic problems in doctor–patient interviews. In *Language and Communication in General Practice* (B. Tanner, ed.), pp. 40–51. Hodder and Stoughton, London.

Davis, M. S. (1966). Variations in patients' compliance with doctors' orders: analysis of congruence between survey responses and results of empirical investigations. *J. Med. Educ.* **41**, 1037–1048.

Davis, M. S. (1968). Variations in patients' compliance with doctors' advice: an experimental analysis of pattern of communication. *Am. J. Public Health* **58**, 274–288.

Di Matteo, M. R., Prince, L. M. and Taranta, A. (1979). Patients' perceptions of physicians' behaviour: determinants of patient commitment to the therapeutic relationship. *J. Comm. Health* **4** (4), 280–290.

Donabedian, A. (1967). Evaluating the quality of medical care. *Milbank Mem. Fund Quart.* **444**, 166–206.

Donabedian, A. (1980). *Explorations in quality assessment and monitoring. Vol. 1: The definition of quality and approaches to its assessment.* Health Administration Press, Ann Arbor, Michigan.

Dorp. C. van (1977). *Luisteren naar Patienten.* De Tijdstroom, Holland.

Dunbar, J. (1979). Issues in assessment. In *New Directions in Patient Compliance.* (S. Cohen, ed.). Lexington Books, New York.

Egbert, L. D., Battit, G. E., Welch, C. E. and Bartlett, M. K. (1964). Reduction of post-operative pain by encouragement and instruction of patients. *New Eng. J. Med.* **270**, 825–827.

Ekman, P., Friesen, W. V. and Ellsworth, P. (1972). *Emotion in the Human Face: Guidelines for Research and an Integration of Findings.* Pergamon Press, New York.

Ellsworth, P. C., Friedman, H. S., Perlick, D. and Hoyt, M. E. (1978). Some effects of gaze on subjects motivated to seek or to avoid social comparison. *J. Exp. Soc. Psychol.* **14**, 69–87.

Fielding, G. and Evered, C. (1978). An exploratory experimental study of the influence of patients' social background upon diagnostic process and outcome. *Psychiatr. Clin. (Base 1)* **11** (2), 61–86.

Ford, J. C. (1977). A linguistic analysis of doctor–patient communication problems: I & II. *Diss. Abst. Inter.* **37** (9A), 5792.

Francis, V., Korsch, B. M. and Morris, M. J. (1969). Gaps in doctor–patient communication: patients' response to medical advice. *New Engl. J. Med.* **280**, 535–540.

Frankel, R. M. (1980). Microanalysis and the medical encounter: an exploratory study. In *Analytic Sociology.* (D. Anderson ed.) Special Edition on Micro-analysis and Medicine.

Freemon, B., Negrete, V. F., Davis, M. and Korsch, B. M. (1971). Gaps in doctor–patient communications: Doctor–patient interaction analysis. *Ped. Res.* **5**, 298–311.

Friedman, H. S. (1979). Nonverbal communication between patients and medical practitioners. *J. Soc. Issues* **35** (1) 82–99.

Friedman, H. S., Di Matteo, M. R. and Taranta, A. (1980). A study of the relationship between individual differences in nonverbal expressiveness and factors of personality and social interaction. *J. Res. Person.* **14**, 351–364.

Gough, H. G. (1977). Doctors' estimates of the percentage of patients whose problems do not require medical attention. *Med. Ed.* **11**, 380–384.

Hays, J. S. and Larsen, K. H. (1963). *Interacting with Patients.* Macmillan, New York.

Henley, B. and Davis, M. S. (1967). Satisfaction and dissatisfaction: a study of the chronically ill aged patient. *J. Health Soc. Behav.* **8**, 65.

Houghton, H. (1968). Problems in hospital communication: an experimental study. In *Problems and Progress in Medical Care: Essays on Current Research. Third Series* (G. McClachlan, ed.). Nuffield Provincial Hospitals Trust, Oxford University Press.

Hugh-Jones, P., Tanser, A. F. and Whitby, C. (1964). Patients' view of admission to a London teaching hospital. *Brit. Med. J.*, **2**, 660–664.

Hulka, B. S., Zyzanski, S. J., Cassel, J. C. *et al.*(1971). Satisfaction with medical care in a low income population. *J. Chron. Dis.* **24**, 661.

Hulka, B. S., Kupper, L. L., Cassel, J. C.and Efird, R. L. (1975). Medication use and misuse: physician–patient discrepancies. *J. Chronic. Dis.* **28** (1), 7–21.

Hulka, B. S., Cassell, J. C., Kuppa, L. L. and Burdette, J. A. (1976). Communication, compliance and concordance between physicians and patients with prescribed medications. *Am. J. Public Health* **66** (9), 847–853.

Hutchinson, J. C. (1979). Hypertension detection and compliance: permanent site hypertensive evaluation—a new method of increasing patient compliance. *Angiology* **30** (8), 568–576.

Irvine, D. H., Webb, J. K. G. and Russell, I. T. (1980). The setting of standards in general practice: research proposal for the development and evaluation of methods, using the care of children in teaching practices in the Northern Region. Unpublished manuscript, Medical Care Research Unit, University of Newcastle-upon-Tyne.

Janis, I. L. (1958). *Psychological Stress: Psychoanalytic and behavioural studies of surgical patients*. Wiley, New York.

Kasl, S. V. (1974). The health belief model and behaviour related to chronic illness. *Health Ed. Monogr.* 2, 433–545.

Kincey, J., Bradshaw, P. and Ley, P. (1975). Patients' satisfaction and reported acceptance of advice in general practice. *J. Roy Coll. Gen. Prac.* 25, 558.

Kirscht, J. P., Becker, M. H., Haefner, D. P. and Maiman, L. P. (1978). Effects of threatening communications and mothers' health beliefs on weight change in obese children. *J. Behav. Med.* 1 (2), 147–157.

Korsch, B. M. and Negrete, V. F. (1972). Doctor–patient communication. *Sci. Amer.* 227 (August), 66–74.

Korsch, B. M., Gozzi, E. K. and Francis, V. (1968). Gaps in doctor–patient communication: 1. Doctor–patient interaction and patient satisfaction. *Pediatrics* 42 (5), 855–871.

Korsch, B. M., Freemon, B. and Negrete, V. F. (1971). Practical implications of doctor–patient interaction: Analysis for pediatric practice. *Am. J. Dis. Children* 121, 110–114.

Krantz, D. S., Baum, A. and Wideman, M. (1980). Assessment of preferences for self-treatment and information in health care. *J. Pers. Soc. Psychol.* 39, 977–990.

Kupst, M. J., Dresser, K., Schulman, J. L. and Paul, M. H. (1975). Evaluation of methods to improve communication in the physician-patient relationship. *Am. J. Orthopsychiatry* 45 (3), 420–429.

Larsen, D. E. and Rootman, I. (1976). Physician role performance and patient satisfaction. *Soc. Sci. Med.* 10, 29–32.

Lebow, J. E. (1974). Consumer assessment of the quality of medical care. *Med. Care* 12, 328–337.

Lewin, K., Dembo, T., Festinger, L. and Sears, P. S. (1944). Level of aspiration. In *Personality and the Behaviour Disorders: A Handbook based on Experimental and Clinical Research* (J. McV. Hunt, ed.). Ronald Press, New York.

Ley, P. (1972). Comprehension, memory and the success of communications with the patient. *J. Inst. Health Ed.* 10, 23–29.

Ley, P. (1976). Towards better doctor–patient communications. In *Communications between Doctors and Patients* (A. E. Bennett ed.). O.U.P. for Nuffield Provincial Hospitals Trust, London.

Ley, P. (1980). *Communication Variables in Health Education*. Health Education Council Monographs, London.

Ley, P., Whitworth, M., Skilbeck, C., Woodward, R., Pinsent, R., Pike, L., Clarkson, M. and Clark, P. (1976). Improving doctor–patient communications in general practice. *J. Roy. Coll. Gen. Prac.* 26, 720–724.

Liptack, G. S., Hulka, B. S. and Cassel, J. C. (1977). Effectiveness of well child care during infancy. *Pediatrics* 60, 186.

Litton-Hawes, E. (1978). A discourse analysis of topic co-selection in medical interviews. *Sociolinguistic Newsletter* 9 (2), 25–26.

Lloyd, M. (1974). Medical authoritarianism and its effect on health care. *Med. J. Aust* 2 (11), 413–416.

Locker, D. and Dunt, D. (1978). Theoretical and methodological issues in sociological studies of consumer satisfaction with medical care. *Soc. Sci. Med.* 12, 283–292.

Long, B. E. L. (1974). Doctors talking to patients: verbal communication. *Gen. Prac. Inter.* 4, 152–158.

Lucas, S. (1978). Health education in general practice: an analysis of information and advice given by doctors in consultations with elderly patients. (Unpublished)

Institute for Social Studies in Medical Care, London.

McAuliffe, W. E. (1978). Studies of process-outcome correlations in medical care evaluations: a critique. *Med. Care* 16, 907–930.

McGhee, A. (1961). *The Patient's Attitude to Nursing Care.* Livingstone, London.

McKinlay, J. B. (1975). Who is really ignorant—physician or patient? *J. Health Soc. Behav.* 16 (1), 3–11.

Marsden, G. (1971). Content analysis studies of psychotherapy: 1954–1968. In *Handbook of Psychotherapy and Behavioural Change* (A. E. Bergin and S. L. Garfield eds)., pp. 345–407. Wiley, N.Y.

Mechanic, D. (1964). The influence of mothers on their children's health behaviour. *Pediatrics* 38, 444.

Mechanic, D. (1974). *Politics, medicine and Social Science.* Wiley, New York.

Melville, A. (1980a). Job satisfaction in general practice: implications for prescribing. *Soc. Sci. Med.* 14A, 495–499.

Melville, K. A. (1980b). Reducing whose anxiety? A Study of the relationship between repeat prescribing of minor tranquillisers and doctors' attitudes. In *Prescribing Practice and Drug Useage* (R. E. A. Mapes, ed.). Croom-Helm, London.

Miller, J. (1978). Diagnosis: a detective story. *The Listener*, 16th November, 640–642.

Miller, S. M. (1980). When is a little information a dangerous thing? Coping with stressful events by monitoring versus blunting. In *Coping and Health* (S. Levine and H. Ursin, eds). Plenum, New York.

Pennebaker, J. W. and Skelton, J. A. (1981). Psychological parameters of physical symptoms. *Pers. Soc. Psych. Bull.* 4, 524–530.

Pietroni, P. (1976). NVC in the G.P. surgery. In *Language and Communication in General Practice.* (B. Tanner, ed), pp. 162–179.

Pratt, L., Seligman, A. and Reader, G. (1957). Physicians' views on the level of information among patients. *Am. J. Pub. Health* 47, 1277.

Pritchard, P. M. P. (1978). *Manual of Primary Health Care.* Oxford University Press, Oxford.

Raimbault, G., Cachin, C., Limal, J. M., Eliacheff, C. and Rappaport, R. (1975). Aspects of communication between patients and doctors: an analysis of the discourse in medical interviews. *Pediatrics* 55 (3), 401–405.

Raynes, N. V. (1980). A preliminary study of search procedures and patient management techniques in general practice. *J. Roy. Coll. Gen. Prac.* 30, 166–172.

Reynolds, M. (1978). No news is bad news: patients' views about communication in hospital. *Brit. Med. J.* (24th June), pp. 1673–1676.

Rhee, San-O (1977). Relative importance of physicians' personal and situational characteristics for the quality of patient care. *J. Health Soc. Behav.* 18, 10–15.

Rieker, P. P. and Begun, J. W. (1980). Translating social science concepts into medical education: a model and curriculum. *Soc. Sci. Med.* 14A, 607–612.

Romm, F. J. and Hulka, B. S. (1979). Care process and patient outcome in diabetes mellitus. *Med. Care* 17 (7), 748–757.

Romm, F. J., Hulka, B. S. and Mayo, F. (1976). Correlates of outcomes in patients with congestive heart failure. *Med. Care* 14, 765.

Rossiter, C. M. Jr. (1975). Defining therapeutic communication. *J. Comm.* 25 (3), 127–130.

Roter, D. L. (1977). Patient participation in the patient-provider interactions: the effects of patient question asking on the quality of interaction, satisfaction and compliance. *Health Ed. Monogr.* 5 (4), 281–315.

RCGP (1972). *The Future General Practitioner: Learning and Teaching.* Royal College of General Practitioners, London.

52   David Pendleton

Scott, R. and Gilmore, M. (1966). The Edinburgh Hospitals. In *Problems and Progress in Medicinal Care* (2nd series). Oxford University Press, Oxford.
Shaw, I. (1976). Consumer opinion and social policy: a research review. *J. Soc. Pol* 5, 19.
Skopek, L. (1979). Doctor–patient conversation: a way of analysing its linguistic problems. *Semiotica* 301–311.
Spelman, M., Ley, P. and Jones, C. (1966). How do we improve doctor–patient communication in our hospitals? *World Hospitals* 2, 126–134.
Stewart, M. A. and Buck, C. W. (1977). Physicians' knowledge of and response to patients' problems. *Med. Care* 15 (7), 578–585.
Stiles, W. B. (1978). Verbal response modes and dimensions of interpersonal roles: a method of discourse analysis. *J. Pers. Soc. Psychol.* 36, 693.
Stiles, W. B., Putnam, S. M., Wolf, M. H. and James, S. A. (1979a). Interaction exchange structure and patient satisfaction with medical interviews. *Med. Care* 17 (6), 667–681.
Stiles, W. B., Putnam, S. M., Wolf, M. H. and James, S. A. (1979b). Verbal response mode profiles of patients and physicians in medical screening interviews. *J. Med. Educ.* 54 (2), 81–89.
Stiles, W. B., Putnam, S. M., James, S. A. and Wolf, M. H. (1979c). Dimensions of patient and physician roles in medical screening interviews. *Soc. Sci. Med.* 13A, 335–341.
Stimson, G. V. (1976). Doctor–patient interaction and some problems for prescribing. *J. Roy. Coll. Gen. Prac.* 26, Suppl. 1, 88–96.
Stimson, G. V. and Webb, B. (1975). *Going to see the Doctor: The Consultation Process in General Practice*. Routledge and Kegan Paul, London.
Tate, P. H. L. (1980). Unpublished data. University of Oxford.
Taylor, S. E. (1979). Hospital patient behaviour: reactance, helplessness or control. *J. Soc. Issues* 35, 156–184.
Truax, C. B. and Carkhuff, R. R. (1967). *Toward Effective Counselling and Psychotherapy: Training and Practice*. Aldine, Chicago.
Truax, C. B. and Mitchell, K. M. (1971). Research on certain therapist interpretation skills in relation to process and outcome. In *Handbook of Psychotherapy and Behavioural Change* (A. E. Bergin and S. L. Garfield, eds). Pp. 299–344. Wiley, New York.
Waitzkin, H. and Stoeckle, J. D. (1972). The communication of information about illness: clinical, social and methodological considerations. *Adv. Psychosom. Med.* 8, 180–215.
Waitzkin, H. and Stoeckle, J. D. (1976). Information control and the micropolitics of health care: summary of an ongoing research project. *Soc. Sci. Med.* 10 (6), 263–276.
Wallston, K. A. and Wallston, B. S. (1978). Preface to the special edition. *Health Education Monogr.* 6 (2), 101–105.
Wallston, B., Wallston, K. and Kaplan, G. (1974 mimeo). Development and validation of the Health Locus of Control (HLC) scale. School of Nursing, Vanderbilt University, Nashville, Tennessee.
Wolf, M. H., Putnam, S. M., James, S. A. and Stiles, W. B. (1978). The medical interview satisfaction scale: development of a scale to measure patient perceptions of physician behaviour. *J. Behav. Med.* 1 (4), 391–401.
Woods, M. M. (1979). Problems in doctor–patient communication: a survey of 100 anaesthetic patients. *Australian Psychologist* 14, 227.
Woolley, F. R., Kane, R. L., Hughes, C. C. and Wright, D. D. (1978). The effects of

doctor–patient communication on satisfaction and outcome of care. *Soc. Sci. Med.* **12** (2A), 123–128.

Wrigglesworth, J. M. and Williams, J. T. (1975). The construction of an objective test to measure patient satisfaction. *Int. J. Nurs. Stud.* **12**, 123–132.

Zola, I. K. (1963). Problems of communication, diagnosis and patient care: the interplay of patient, physician and clinic organization. *J. Med. Ed.* **38**, 829–838.

Zola, I. K. (1972). Studying the decision to see a doctor: review, critique, corrective. In *Psychological Aspects of Physical Illness*. Vol. 8 in *Advances in Psychosomatic Medicine* (Z. J. Lipowski, ed.). Karger, Basel.

Zyzanski, S. J., Hulka, B. S. and Cassel, J. C. (1974). Scale for measurement of "Satisfaction" with medical care: modifications in content, format and scoring. *Med. Care* **12**, 611.

Part 1
Behaviour in the Consultation

2 Doctor–Patient Skills

Michael Argyle

1 SOCIAL SKILLS AND SOCIAL COMPETENCE

The work of doctors is like that of teachers, managers, social workers, and many others, in that their work consists of dealing with people. In each case technical knowledge and skills are required, but this cannot be used unless the practitioner is able to communicate, persuade, and generally deal with his clients. Some of the earliest studies of social skills were carried out on supervisors of working groups. It was found that the supervisors who used certain styles of supervision had groups which produced twice as much, or had one eighth the rate of absenteeism or labour turnover, as those of other supervisors (Argyle, 1972). Similar figures can be given for selling, where again there is a simple index of social effectiveness. These studies demonstrate clearly that differences in social skill, i.e. style of social performance, have a great influence on overall effectiveness.

It is fairly easy to measure the success of a salesman—by the amount of goods sold, over a period, in relation to the average for other salesmen in a similar selling situation. How can the success of doctors be assessed? It depends on what are thought to be the goals of a doctor. The average level of health of his patients is the ultimate criterion, but no-one has attempted to measure this; in any case it would depend on the kind of patients in the practice. The recovery rate of ill patients who have been seen is another possibility, and this is more feasible. Objective indices which have been used include number of days needed in hospital after an operation, and memory for and compliance with the doctor's instructions. If the subjective state of patients is regarded as important, ratings of patient satisfaction could be used. (Chapter 1 reviews the available literature on measurements of outcomes of care.) Another approach is to make use of ratings by professional colleagues, who have seen a doctor at work, or have observed him in role-played clinical situations dealing with standardized problems.

The next step is to discover the most effective social skills, so that they can be taught to practitioners. A number of studies of supervisory skills compared the styles of behaviour used by good and bad supervisors, i.e. those in charge of high and low output work teams. This kind of research led to the discovery of the optimum supervisory skills—though these were found to vary somewhat with the situation (Argyle, op. cit.). In the case of cross-cultural interaction skills a different approach has been used— carrying out critical incident surveys of large numbers of instances where, for example, Americans got into difficulties with Arabs. These instances were classified into their main groups, experts advised on where those involved went wrong, and training materials were devised accordingly as described by Brislin and Pedersen (1976). However, social competence has many components, some of them rather subtle, and it is necessary to have some understanding of these components in order to anticipate and understand the possible sources of success and failure in social skills.

When the optimum social skills have been discovered, the final step is to train practitioners to use them. In the early days of the study of social skills it was thought that lecture and discussion methods would do the job, but it soon became clear that this was not so. Specialized forms of role-playing and related methods have been devised and follow-up studies conducted. The most effective methods of social skills training (SST) will be described later.

2 THE SOCIAL SKILL MODEL

We can look at social behaviour as a skilled performance similar to motor skills like driving a car (see Fig. 2.1.)

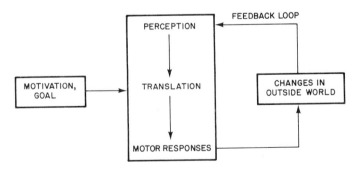

Fig. 2.1.   Motor skill model (from Argyle, 1967).

In each case the performer is pursuing certain goals, makes continuous response to feedback and emits hierarchically-organized motor responses. This model has been heuristically very useful in drawing attention to the importance of feedback, and hence to gaze; it also suggests a number of different ways in which social performances can fail, and suggests the training procedures that may be effective, through analogy with motor skills training (Argyle and Kendon, 1967 and Argyle, 1969).

The model emphasizes the motivation, goals and plans of interactors. It is postulated that every interactor is trying to achieve some goal, whether he is aware of it or not. These goals may be for example to get another person to like him, to obtain or convey information, to modify the other's emotional state, and so on. Such goals may be linked to more basic motivational systems. Goals have sub-goals: for example a doctor may have to diagnose the patient before he can treat him. Patterns of response are directed towards goals and sub-goals, and have a hierarchical structure—large units of behaviour are composed of smaller ones, and at the lowest levels these are habitual and automatic.

Harré and Secord (1972) have argued persuasively that much human social behaviour is the result of conscious planning, often in words, with full regard for the complex meanings of behaviour, and the rules of situations. This is an important correction to earlier social psychological views, which often failed to recognize the complexity of individual planning and the different meanings which may be given to stimuli, for example in laboratory experiments. However, it must be recognized that much social behaviour is *not* planned in this way: the smaller elements of behaviour and longer automatic sequences are outside conscious awareness, though it is possible to attend for example to patterns of gaze, shifts of orientation, or the latent meanings of utterances. The social skill model, in emphasizing the hierarchical structure of social performance, can incorporate both kinds of behaviour.

The social skill model also emphasizes feedback processes. A person driving a car sees at once when it is going in the wrong direction, and takes corrective action with the steering wheel. Social interactors do likewise—if another person is talking too much they interrupt, ask closed questions or no questions, and look less interested in what he has to say. Feedback requires perception, looking at and listening to the other person. Skilled performance requires the ability to take the appropriate corrective action referred to as "translation" in the model—not everyone knows that open-ended questions make people talk more and closed questions make them talk less. The social skills which are most effective vary with the situation and the other persons present. Patients of different age, sex, class, and personality will need to be handled differently. The details of such variation in skill will require a lot of research before they are fully mapped out.

2.1 The Role of Reinforcement

This is one of the key processes in social skill sequences. When interactor A does what B wants him to do, B is pleased and sends immediate and spontaneous reinforcements—smile, gaze, approving noises, etc. and modifies A's behaviour, probably by operant conditioning—for example modifying what he says. At the same time A is modifying B's behaviour in exactly the same way. These effects appear to be mainly outside the focus of conscious attention, and take place very rapidly. It follows that anyone who gives strong rewards and punishments in the course of interaction will be able to modify the behaviour of others in the desired direction. In addition, the stronger the *rewards* that A issues, the more strongly other people will be attracted to him.

2.2. The Role of Gaze in Social Skills

The social skill model suggests that the monitoring of another's reactions is an essential part of social performance. The other's verbal signals are mainly heard, but his non-verbal signals are mainly seen—the exceptions being the non-verbal aspects of speech, and touch. It was this implication of the social skill model which directed us towards the study of gaze in social interaction. In interaction between two people each person looks about 50% of the time, mutual gaze occupies up to 25% of the time, looking while listening is about twice the level of looking while talking, glances are about 3 sec, and mutual glances about 1 sec, with wide variations due to distance, sex combinations and personality (Argyle and Cook, 1976).

However, there are several important differences between social behaviour and motor skills.

2.2.1 *Rules*

The moves which interactors may make are governed by rules—they must respond properly to what has gone before. Similarly rules govern the other's responses and can be used to influence his behaviour, e.g. questions usually lead to answers.

2.2.2 *Taking the role of the other*

It is important to perceive accurately the reactions of others. It is also necessary to perceive the perceptions of others, i.e. to take account of their point of view. This appears to be a cognitive ability which develops with age (Flavell 1968), but which may fail to develop properly. Those who are able to do this have been found to be more effective at a number of social tasks, and more altruistic. Meldman (1967) found that psychiatric patients were more egocentric, i.e. talked about themselves more than controls, and it has been our experience that socially unskilled patients have great difficulty in taking the role of the other.

2.3 The independent initiative of the other—sequences of interaction

Social situations inevitably contain at least one other person, who will be pursuing *his* goals and using *his* social skills. How can we analyse the resulting sequences of behaviour? For a sequence to constitute an acceptable piece of social behaviour, the moves must fit together in order. We shall discuss the properties of sequences of interaction later.

3 VERBAL AND NON-VERBAL COMMUNICATIONS

One of the main components of socially skilled performance is verbal communication—though we shall see that it is closely supported by non-verbal communication (NVC). In some situations skilled behaviour simply involves more speech, but usually it is the detailed performance of tactful, persuasive or otherwise effective utterances which are important. The details of these in the case of doctors are discussed elsewhere (see Chapter 1, this volume).

There are several different kinds of verbal utterance:

(a) *Egocentric speech* is directed to the self, is found in infants and has the effect of directing one's behaviour.

(b) *Orders, instructions,* are used to influence the behaviour of others; they can be gently persuasive or authoritarian.

(c) *Questions* are intended to elicit verbal information; they can be open-ended or closed, personal or impersonal.

(d) *Information* may be given in response to a question, as part of a lecture, or during problem-solving discussion.

(e) *Informal speech,* consists of casual chat, jokes, gossip, and contains little information, but helps to establish and sustain social relationships.

(f) *Expression of emotions and interpersonal attitudes.* This is a special kind of information; however as we shall see, this information is usually conveyed and is conveyed more effectively non-verbally.

(g) *"Performative" utterances.* These include "illocutions" where saying the

utterance performs something (voting, judging, naming, etc.), and "per-
locutions", where a goal is intended though it may not be achieved
(persuading, intimidating, etc.).

(h) *Social routines* include standard sequences like thanking, apologising,
greeting, etc.

(i) *Latent messages* are where the more important meaning is made subordinate
("As I was saying to the Prime Minister . . .").

Byrne and Long (op. cit.) have suggested a very long repertoire for doctors,
but shorter sets of categories have also been devised. It remains to be seen
which set of categories captures most usefully the essential behaviour of
doctors, discriminates between effective and less effective doctors, and is
found to be most useful in training.

3.1 Non-Verbal Signals Accompanying Speech

Non-verbal signals also play an important part in speech, and conversation.
They have three main roles:

3.1.1 *Completing and elaborating on verbal utterances*

Some utterances are meaningless or ambiguous unless the NV accompaniments are taken into account. A lecturer may point at part of a diagram: a
tape-recording of this part of the lecture would be meaningless. Some
sentences are ambiguous if printed—"They are hunting dogs", but not if
spoken—"they are hunting *dogs*". Gestural illustrations are used to amplify
the meaning of utterances, and succeed in doing so. The way in which an
utterance is delivered "frames" it, i.e. the intonation and facial expression
indicate whether it is intended to be serious, and so on; the NV accompani-
ment is a message about the message, which is needed by the recipient in order
to know what to do with it.

3.1.2 *Managing synchronizing*

When two or more people are talking they have to take turns to speak. This
is achieved mainly by means of NV signals. For example if a speaker wants to
avoid being interrupted, he will be more successful if he does not look up at the
ends of sentences, keeps a hand in mid-gesture at these points, and if, when
interrupted, he immediately increases the loudness of his speech. It has been
found that completing a clause and change in pitch-level are important signals
for indicating the end of an utterance. A question combined with prolonged
gaze is another (Beattie, 1980).

3.1.3 *Sending feedback signals*

When someone is speaking he needs intermittent, but regular, feedback on how others are responding, so that he can modify his utterances accordingly. He needs to know whether the listeners understand, believe or disbelieve, are surprised or bored, agree or disagree, are pleased or annoyed. This information could be provided by *sotto voce* verbal muttering on their part, but is in fact obtained by careful study of their faces: the eyebrows signal surprise, puzzlement, etc., while the mouth indicates pleasure and displeasure. When the other is invisible, as in telephone conversation, these visual signals are unavailable, and more verbalized "listening behaviour" is used—"I see", "really?", "how interesting", etc.

3.2 Other functions of Non-Verbal Communication (NVC)

Non-verbal communication is a very important component of social skill. Several studies have shown that successful interactors smile more, look more and have different intonation. NVC consists mainly of facial expression, tone of voice, gaze, gestures, postures, physical proximity and appearance. We have already described how NVC is linked with speech; it also functions in several other ways, especially in the communication of emotions and attitudes to other people.

A *sender* is in a certain state, or possesses some information; this is *encoded* into a message which is then *decoded* by a *receiver*.

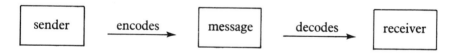

Encoding research is done by putting subjects into some state and studying the NV messages which are emitted. For example Mehrabian (1968) in a role-played experiment, asked subject to address a hat-stand, imagining it to be a person. Male subjects who liked the hat-stand looked at it more, did not have hands on hips and stood closer.

3.2.1 *Interpersonal attitudes*

We are concerned here with attitudes towards others who are present. The main attitudes fall along two dimensions:

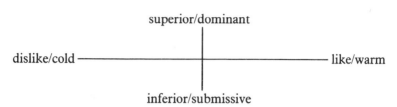

In addition there is love, which is a variant of like. These attitudes can be conveyed clearly by non-verbal signals, such as facial expression, tone of voice and posture. Liking is conveyed by smiling, a friendly tone of voice and so on.

The author and his colleagues compared the affect of verbal and non-verbal signals for communicating interpersonal attitudes. It was found that the variance due to non-verbal cues was about 12 times the variance due to verbal cues, in affecting judgements of inferior-superior (Argyle *et al.*, 1970).

4 SEQUENCES OF SOCIAL INTERACTION

Social psychologists have not yet discovered all the principles or "grammar" underlying these sequences, but some of the principles are known, and can explain common forms of interaction failure.

4.1 Two-Step Sequences

Conversational sequences are partly constructed out of certain basic building blocks, like the question–answer sequence, and repeated cycles characteristic of the situation. Socially inadequate people are usually very bad conversationalists and this appears to be due to a failure to master some of these basic sequences.

There are a number of other common 2-step sequences such as joke–laugh, complain–sympathize, request–comply or refuse. There are a number of 2-step sequences which take place not because there is a rule, but as a result of basic psychological processes. For example there is the powerful effect of re-inforcement, and there is response-matching, in which one person copies the accent, posture or other aspects of the other's behaviour.

There are also *pro-active* 2-step sequences, where one person makes both moves, as in accept–thank, reply–question. Failure to make a pro-active move can stop a conversation, as in this example:

A.   Where do you come from?
B.   Swindon
      (end of conversation)

B should have used a double, or "pro-active" move, of the type, "I come from Swindon; where do *you* come from?"

These reactive and pro-active 2-step pairs can build up to make repeated cycles, as happens in the classroom:

Teacher: lectures
Teacher: asks questions
Pupil: replies
Teacher: comments
(cycle repeats). (After Flanders, 1970.)

4.2 Social Skill Sequences

We turn now to sequences longer than 2 steps. The social skill model generates a characteristic kind of 4-step sequence:

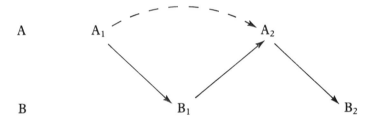

this is a case of asymmetrical contingency, with A in charge. A's first move A_1 produces an unsatisfactory result, B_1, so A modifies his behaviour to A_2, which produces the desired B_2. Note the links A_1–A_2, representing the persistence of A's goal-directed behaviour. This can be seen in the social survey interview:

I_1: asks question
R_1: gives inadequate answer, or does not understand question
I_2: clarifies and repeats question
R_2: gives adequate answer

Teachers and interviewers, like doctors, are more or less in charge of the situation; their clients have much less control and initiative, and largely respond to the doctor's instructions. These are all cases of "asymmetrical interaction".

4.3 Episode sequence

Most social encounters consist of a number of distinct episodes, which may have come in a particular order. It has been suggested by Byrne and Long (1976) that doctor–patient encounters contain six main episodes, which usually come in a certain order, though not all will be present on a particular occasion:

(1) relating to the patient
(2) discussing the reason for the patient's attendance
(3) conducting a verbal or physical examination or both
(4) consideration of patient's condition
(5) detailing treatment or further investigation
(6) terminating

They found that all six phases occurred in only 63% of interviews, and that sometimes part of the sequence was repeated.

The task in turn may consist of several sub-tasks, e.g. a doctor has to conduct a verbal or physical examination—make a diagnosis—carry out or prescribe treatment. Often, as in this case, the sub-tasks have to come in a certain order. At primarily social events the "task" seems to consist of eating or drinking accompanied by the exchange of information.

5 SITUATIONS, THEIR RULES AND OTHER FEATURES

The traditional trait model supposed that individuals possess a fixed degree of introversion, neuroticism etc., and that it is displayed consistently in different situations. This model has been abandoned by most psychologists following an increased awareness of the great effect of the situation on behaviour (e.g. people are more anxious when exposed to physical danger than when asleep in bed), and the amount of person–situation interaction (e.g. person A is more frightened by heights, B by cows), resulting in low inter-situational consistency (Mischel, 1968).

A long series of studies attempted to test trait theory and other models by finding the percentages of variance due to persons, situations and P × S interaction. This was done with reported behaviour (e.g. anxiety), and with observed behaviour (e.g. talking, smiling). Typical results were:

persons	15–30%
situations	20–45%
P × S	30–50%

[Unfortunately it is not possible to give any exact figures, since there is no way of producing equivalent degrees of variation of personality and situation (Endler and Magnusson, 1976).] These results show that a simple trait theory must be abandoned. The alternative position which has developed is known as interactionism, which recognizes the independent contribution of persons, situations and interactions between them, and accepts that the detailed prediction of behaviour requires equations of the form $B = f(P,S)$.

However, the interactionist model has a number of serious limitations. (1) Persons choose the situations in which they are found, and avoid others, so P has two different effects. (2) Persons can, to some extent, change the situation they are in, for example generating friendly or hostile behaviour from others. (3) Although some behaviour occurs in all situations, e.g. level of anxiety and amount of talk, situations also have repertoires of behaviour which are unique to them—the moves of chess are different from those of football. The interactionist equations cannot be applied here. (4) There are problems about specifying the dimensions of situations to enter into the equation, as will be shown below.

Whether we adopt the interactionist position or some other we need to be able to measure or assess situations. We suggest that the most useful way of doing this is to describe their main features, just as one might describe a game in terms of its rules, physical setting, how to win, and so on. The main features appear to be as follows:

5.1 Goals

In all situations there are certain goals which are commonly obtainable. It is often fairly obvious what these are, but socially inadequate people may simply not know what parties are for, for example, or may think that the purpose of a selection interview is vocational guidance.

We have studied the main goals in a number of common situations, by asking samples of people to rate the importance of various goals, and then carrying out factor analyses. The main goals are usually (1) social acceptance etc, (2) food, drink and other bodily needs, (3) task goals specific to the situation. We have also studied the relations between goals, within and between persons, in terms of conflict and instrumentality. This makes it possible to study the "goal structure" of situations. An example from Graham *et al.* (1981) is given in Fig. 5.2 showing that the only conflict between nurses and patients is between the nurses' concern for the bodily well-being of the patients and of themselves.

5.2 Rules

All situations have rules about what may or may not be done in them. Socially inadequate people are often ignorant or mistaken about the rules. It

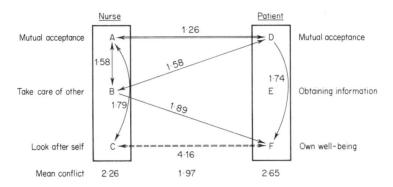

Fig. 2.2   Nurse–Patient goal structure (conflict rated 1–5).

would obviously be impossible to play a game without knowing the rules and the same applies to social situations.

We have studied the rules of a number of everyday situations. There appear to be several universal rules—be polite, be friendly, do not embarrass people. There are also rules which are specific to situations, since they enable situational goals to be met. We have found that patients consider that there are rules which apply to them when visiting the doctor—make sure your body is clean and tell the truth. Pendleton has found that there are rules which patients consider apply to doctors—(See Chapter 7, this volume.)

5.3 Special Skills

Many social situations require special social skills, as in the case of various kinds of public speaking and interviewing, but also such everyday situations as dates and parties. A person with little experience of a particular situation may find that he lacks the special skills needed for it (cf. Argyle *et al.*, 1981). This particularly applies to professional skills such as those needed by doctors.

5.4 Repertoire of Elements

Every situation defines certain moves as relevant. For example, at a seminar it is relevant to show slides, make long speeches, draw on the blackboard etc. If moves appropriate to a cricket match or a Scottish ball were made, they would be ignored or regarded as totally bizarre.

5.5 Roles

Every situation has a limited number of roles, e.g. a classroom has the roles of teacher, pupil, janitor and school inspector. These roles carry different degrees of power, and the occupant has goals peculiar to that role.

5.6 Cognitive Structure

We found that the members of a research group classified each other in terms of the concepts *extraverted* and *enjoyable companion* for social occasions. Performers of professional social skills classify their clients in ways related to the task. It is very likely that doctors classify their patients in terms of health and type of illness, but perhaps they also separate out those who need to be handled differently.

5.7 Environmental Setting and Pieces

Most situations involve special environmental settings and props. Cricket needs bat, ball, stumps etc.; a seminar requires blackboard, slide projector and lecture notes. Doctors have their special settings too, though there is quite a lot of variation between the equipment and furnishings displayed by different kinds of doctor.

6 SELF-PRESENTATION

During social interaction people form impressions of one another, including how good others are at their job. It is also possible to manipulate the impressions which are formed by others, and this is known as "self-presentation". This is done partly to sustain self-esteem, and partly for professional purposes—teachers teach more effectively if their pupils think they are well-informed, for example. It is very likely that patients recover faster if they are confident that the doctor can cure them, particularly in the case of mental patients.

How is self-presentation done? If people tell others how good they are in words, this is regarded as a joke and disbelieved, in Western cultures at least. E. E. Jones (1964) found that verbal ingratiation is done with subtlety—drawing attention to assets in unimportant areas for example. Most self-presentation is done non-verbally—by clothes, hair-style, accent, badges and general style of behaviour. Social class is very clearly signalled in these ways, as is membership of rebellious social groups (Argyle, 1975).

Goffman (1956) maintained that social behaviour involves a great deal of deceptive self-presentation, by individuals and groups, which is often in the interest of those deceived as in the work of morticians and doctors. In everyday life, deception is probably less common than concealment. Most people keep quiet about discreditable events in their past, and others do not remind them. Stigmatized individuals like homosexuals, drug-addicts and members of certain professions also keep it dark, though they are usually recognized by other members. Goffman's theory gives an explanation of embarrassment —this occurs when false self-presentation is unmasked. Later research demonstrated that this was so, but that embarrassment also occurs when other people break social rules, and when social accidents are committed—unintentional *gaffes*, and forgetting names, for example (Argyle, 1969).

Physical attractiveness is partly a matter of self-presentation, inasmuch as it is partly, even mainly, under an individual's control. Attention to clothes, hair and skin, dieting, facial expression and posture, can do a great deal to modify physical attractiveness. People who are attractive are believed to be better in all sorts of ways, are liked more, according to Berscheid and Walster (1973), and as a result are probably more effective at their jobs. It is also very important that a professional social skill performer should have an appropriate appearance for his role—it is no good a doctor looking, for example, like a mad scientist or a down and out.

7 TRAINING IN SOCIAL SKILLS

7.1 Role-playing, with Coaching

This is now the most widely-used method of SST. There are four stages: (a) instruction, (b) role-playing with other trainees or other role partners for 5–8 min, (c) feedback and coaching, in the form of verbal comments from the trainer, (d) repeated role-playing. A typical laboratory set-up is shown in Fig 2·3 here. This also shows the use of an ear-microphone, for instruction while role-playing is taking place.

For an individual or group of trainees, a series of topics, skills or situations is chosen, and introduced by means of short scenarios. Role partners are used, who can be briefed to present carefully graded degrees of difficulty.

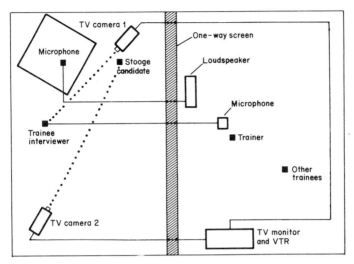

Fig. 2.3.   Social skills training laboratory.

It is usual for trainers to be generally encouraging, and also rewarding for specific aspects of behaviour, though there is little experimental evidence for the value of such reinforcement. It is common to combine role-playing with modelling and video play-back, both of which are discussed below.

7.1.1 *Modelling*

This can consist of demonstrations by one of the trainers, or showing films or video-tapes of an experienced practitioner at work. It is generally used in conjunction with role-playing, between role-play sessions, and is accompanied by verbal instructions, i.e. coaching.

7.1.2 *Video play-back*

This is widely used in conjunction with role-playing. Bailey and Sowder (1970) and Griffiths (1974) have reviewed some of the studies comparing the effectiveness of role-playing with and without video, and come to the conclusion that there is little evidence for its usefulness. In fact nearly all the studies cited showed that trainees did better when video playback was used. A later carefully-designed study by Maxwell (1976), on people who replied to an advertisement for SST, obtained clearly better results with video; the criterion measure consisted of "blind" ratings of role-playing. Most people find it mildly disturbing at first, and that it increases self-consciousness; however, this wears off by the second or third session. The author has found it particularly useful in training non-verbal behaviour.

7.1.3 *"Homework"*

How do trainees apply what they have learned in the training setting to real life situations? The main solution so far has been via "homework". Trainees are asked to try out the skills which they have just learnt several times before the next weekly session, and to report back on any difficulties. They may be given written notes on the exercises to be carried out, and the steps involved in each, and they may be asked to keep notes of what happened. Falloon (1977) found that out-patients who were given structured homework assignments did better on nearly all outcome measures.

7.1.4 *Individual vs group methods*

It is usual to carry out SST for professional people in groups of about six. This has the advantage of economizing on trainer time, and of providing role-partners. On the other hand role-playing has been found to be more successful if genuine clients are provided.

Some forms of SST have drawn heavily on the results of research in social psychology, and this is particularly the case with the Oxford form of SST. Here are some examples, related to the processes described earlier.

(*a*) *Expression of NVC.* People who are unable to express emotions and interpersonal attitudes can be given training in the use of the face and voice. Facial expression can be taught with the help of a mirror, and then a video-tape-recorder; vocal expression training needs an audio tape-recorder.

(*b*) *Situational analysis.* For clients who have difficulty with particular situations, situational analysis is useful. The goals, rules, repertoire, roles, and other features of the situation are established, the difficulties located, and the best solutions are discussed and practised.

(*c*) *Analysis of conversational sequences.* Some people cannot sustain a simple conversation. Study of their social performance in role-playing sessions makes it possible to discover exactly what it is they are doing wrong—e.g. failure to reciprocate or hand over conversation, failure of non-verbal accompaniments, etc. Coaching is then directed towards these deficits.

(*d*) *Perceptual training.* Doctors become skilled in the observation of bodies, and can tell a lot from what is visible. These perceptual skills can be extended to include the accurate perception of anxiety or other emotions, from face and voice, and the site and type of pains by the gestures used to describe them.

7.2 Other Methods of Training

7.2.1 *Training on the job*

This is a widely-used traditional method. Some people improve through supervision but others do not, and some learn the wrong things. The situation can be improved if there is a trainer who regularly sees the trainee in action, and is able to hold feedback sessions at which errors are pointed out and better skills suggested. In practice this method does not appear to work very well, for example with trainee teachers (see Argyle, 1969).

7.2.2 *Group methods*

Group methods, especially T-groups, are intended to enhance sensitivity and social skills. Follow-up studies have consistently found that 30–40% of trainees are improved by group methods, but up to 10% are worse, sometimes needing psychological assistance (e.g. Lieberman *et al.*, 1973). It has been argued that group methods are useful for those who are resistant to being trained. Group methods are sometimes used with medical students or young doctors in the hope that they may promote "personal growth"— giving students the self-confidence and the capacity to deal with difficult emotional, ethical or legal problems, with matters of life and death. A better course would perhaps be group discussions led by experienced practitioners, at which these problems can be aired.

7.2.3 *Educational methods*

Educational methods such as lectures and films, can increase knowledge, but to master social skills it is necessary to try them out, as is the case with motor skills. Educational methods can be a useful supplement to role-playing methods. They have been found particularly useful in training people for inter-cultural skills, probably because there is a lot to be learnt about the rules and ideas of the other culture (Brislin and Pedersen, 1976).

REFERENCES

Argyle, M. (1969). *Social Interaction*. Methuen, London.
Argyle, M. (1972). *The Social Psychology of Work*. Allen Lane the Penguin Press, London.

Argyle, M. and Cook, M. (1976). *Gaze and Mutual Gaze.* Cambridge University Press, Cambridge.

Argyle, M. and Kendon, A. (1967). The experimental analysis of social performance. *Adv. Exp. Soc. Psychol.* **3**, 55–98.

Argyle M., Salter, V., Nicholson, H., Williams, M. and Burgess, P. (1970). The communication of inferior and superior attitudes by verbal and non-verbal signals. *Brit. Jo. Soc. Clin. Psychol.* **9**, 221–231.

Argyle, M., Furnham, A. and Graham, J. A. (1981). *Social Situations.* Cambridge University Press, Cambridge.

Bailey, K. G. and Sowder, W. T. (1970). Audiotape and videotape self-confrontation in psychotherapy. *Psychol. Bull.* **74**, 127–137.

Beattie, G. W. (1980). The skilled art of conversational interaction: verbal and non-verbal signals in its regulation and management. In *The Analysis of Social Skill* (W. T. Singleton *et al.*, eds), pp. 193–211. Plenum, New York and London.

Berscheid, E. and Walster, E. H. (1973). Physical attractiveness. In *Advances in Experimental Social Psychology*, Vol. 7 (L. Berkowitz, ed.). Academic Press, New York.

Brislin, R. W. and Pedersen, P. (1976). *Cross-Cultural Orientation Programs.* Gardner Press, New York.

Byrne, P. and Long, B. E. L. (1976). *Doctors Talking to Patients.* H.M.S.O., London.

Ekman, P., Friesen, W. V. and Ellsworth, P. (1972). *Emotion in the Human Face.* Pergamon Press, New York.

Falloon, I. R. H., Lindley, P., McDonald, R. and Marks, I. M. (1977). Social skills training of out-patient groups: a controlled study of rehearsal and homework. *Brit. J. Psychiat.* **131**, 599–609.

Flanders, N. A. (1970). *Analyzing Teaching Behavior.* Addison-Wesley, Massachusetts.

Flavell, J. H. (1968). *The Development of Role-taking and Communication Skills in Children.* Wiley, New York.

Goffman, E. (1956). *The Presentation of Self in Everyday Life.* Edinburgh University Press, Edinburgh.

Graham, J. A., Argyle, M. and Furnham, A. (1980). The goal structure of situations. *Eur. J. Soc. Psychol.* **10**, 345–366.

Griffiths, R. D. P. (1974). Videotape feedback as a therapeutic technique: retrospect and prospect. *Behav. Res. Ther.* **12**, 1–8.

Harré, R. and Secord, P. (1972). *The Explanation of Social Behaviour.* Blackwell, Oxford.

Jones, E. E. (1964). *Ingratiation: a Social Psychological Analysis.* Appleton-Century-Crofts, New York.

Lieberman, M. A., Yalom, I. D. and Miles, M. R. (1973). *Encounter Groups: First Facts.* Basic Books, New York.

Maxwell, G. M. (1976). An evaluation of social skills training. Unpublished. University of Otago, Dunedin, New Zealand.

Mehrabian, A. (1972). *Nonverbal Communication.* Aldine-Atherton, Chicago and New York.

Meldman, M. J. (1967). Verbal behavior analysis of self-hyperattentionism. *Dis. Nerv. System* **28**, 469–473.

Mischel, W. (1968). *Personality and Assessment.* Wiley, New York.

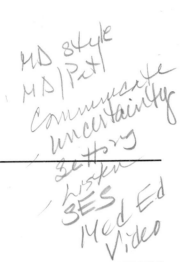

3   Doctors' Style

Peter Tate

That doctors differ considerably in their approach to the practice of medicine is self-evident. It is the reasons for and the effects of these differences that are so interesting and ultimately so important in the future training of General Practitioners.

A doctor's style is an amalgam of behaviours derived from his personal beliefs, knowledge, experience and skilfulness. The individual variations are infinite but certain broad categories are recognizable. In their large study of consultations in general practice, entitled "Doctors talking to patients", Byrne and Long (1976) described the range of behaviours exhibited on a scale ranging from doctor-centred to patient-centred. The majority of doctors practice toward the doctor-centred end of this spectrum, which is the traditional authoritarian approach based on the assumption that the doctor is responsible for his patient's health and will go through his agenda for the patient. At the other end of the scale, the doctor is seen as much less authoritarian, the responsibility for health is shared and the patient is encouraged to go through his own agenda not the doctor's.

1 REASONS FOR ADOPTING A STYLE

Most doctors have never been trained to consult in a general practice setting. The traditional clinical history taking model is too cumbersome and, early in their careers, doctors collect together groups of behaviours according to their skills and experience and begin repeating these day after day. The fact that their experience at this stage is almost totally based on skills acquired in large teaching hospitals, makes it unsurprising that the patterns of behaviour tend to be disease-orientated and self-protectively authoritarian.

For a young partner in General Practice, it is hard to discern the effect of the various strategies adopted, and the patterns soon become fixed.

A doctor's attitudes are clearly reflected in the way he deals with patients but these attitudes are also related to his skilfulness. For example, if he is unskilled in counselling techniques, he is likely to rely on rather authoritative pronouncements and feel that counselling is the province of other disciplines. But, if, by training, he acquired some skills of counselling, his attitude is likely to be modified. It requires special skills to interview and listen to patients.

2 FLEXIBILITY OF STYLE

There is evidence from Byrne and Long (1976) and Bloor (1978) that, when doctors have developed a set of behaviours, they use these stock patterns again and again and that many of these behaviours are not significantly influenced by the patient's presenting problem. Raynes (1980) suggests that prescribing seems to be one of these activities. This inherent lack of flexibility was demonstrated clearly by Byrne and Long (1976). Using a detailed scoring system, they graded doctors' behaviour into categories between doctor- and patient-centred. They found that doctors remained in these categories consistently for a wide variety of patients with only limited movements across the spectrum. No doctor appeared to span the whole range; those described as patient-centred showed more flexibility but the overall results show a chastening rigidity.

Future training for general practice must concentrate on communication. Increasing the number of such skills a doctor possesses will increase his capacity for flexibility. This, in turn, may well influence his attitudes.

3 STYLE RELATED TO AUTHORITY

The effects of varying styles of behaviours can be represented diagrammatically. The left hand side shows the large doctor contribution, with relatively small input from the patient, and, towards the right hand side, the position is reversed. This sort of diagram is known as a "power shift model" and that is exactly what it demonstrates.

The power society invests in its doctors is a fascinating field for study. Each individual doctor's need for power is probably one of the main guiding factors in the manner in which he practices medicine. When discussing power in this context I mean both authority and the ability to influence, particularly in relation to the reduction of anxiety.

The traditional authoritarian approach adopted by the majority of doctors is

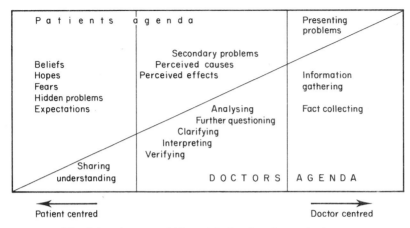

Fig. 3.1. A power shift model of styles of consultation.

a powerful model and is also the style most expected by patients according to Fitton and Acheson (1979). On the other hand, the sharing and listening approach probably decreases some of the doctor's authority and, although understanding in the patient is increased, perhaps the magical healing and anxiety relieving power is actually reduced. This is an equation that needs to be investigated thoroughly. If future training is to advocate more skilful sharing but less powerful ways of communication, the consequent increase in self-responsibility and understanding must outweigh the decrease in comforting and anxiety relieving. It is probably not within an individual doctor's capability to come completely off the hill that society sets him upon but he must learn to be aware of the profit and losses entailed by striving to be closer to his patients.

Another definition of doctor power relates to the doctor's ability to increase his own certainty while maintaining some uncertainty in the patient described by Waitzkin and Stoekle (1972). The definition states that a physician's ability to preserve his own power in the doctor–patient relationship depends largely on the ability to control the patient's uncertainty. The implication here is that the instructing and advising approach, without meaningful explanations, retains the doctor as a powerful figure; when information is shared the doctor will reduce some of his powerfulness. Doctors who wish to have a lot of influence over their patients may thus consciously or unconsciously maintain a degree of uncertainty.

Medical authority has been defined by Osmond (1980) as consisting of three parts, sapiental, moral and charismatic:

(a) Sapiental authority is the right to be heard derived from knowledge or expertise. In other words, doctors must know or appear to know more about medicine than their patients.

(b) Moral authority is the right to control and direct based on doing what is expected of them as doctors and their concern with the good of the patient.

(c) The third, and by far the most difficult, is charismatic authority; the right to control and direct that is derived from God-given grace. This threesome has been called "Aesculapian authority". The charismatic authority, in this definition, comes close to the use of magic as defined by anthropologists. Patients are aware that medicine deals with powerful and mysterious forces not completely amenable to reason. Life and death are arbitrary, so it is not surprising that doctors are invested with the ability to relieve suffering and fear by means that are not strictly scientific or even rational.

Ever since man formed groups the healers have been invested with special powers and most healing has been brought about by anxiety reduction produced by powerful suggestion. Tribes have used this sort of magic. Sacrifices to appease the gods may or may not have that effect but will certainly reduce the anxiety in the tribe. Similarly, with the rain dance, it may not bring rain but temporarily the tribe will be less anxious. If a powerful healer tells the patient he will recover and mixes this with ritual the patient immediately feels better and perhaps more able to cope with real as well as imagined disease.

This argument may sound a long way from a Friday afternoon surgery but the doctor sitting behind his desk questioning and then firmly giving advice is achieving some of his therapeutic aims by using his charismatic authority. As he is seen as a healer his words have the power to reduce anxiety and reassure, even if the scientific content of the message is suspect. This is not a placebo effect; this is an effect of the power which is invested in him by the patient and society. Doctors can encourage or discourage their patients to see them as authority figures in many ways, seating positions and dress are just two examples. Doctors who sit behind their desk maintain a rigid distance between themselves and their patients. Every business executive is aware of the maintaining of power differentials by this method.

4 SEATING POSITION

Behavioural studies show (Pietroni, 1976) that the position in which the doctor sits in relation to the patient profoundly influences the mutual exchange (Fig. 3.2).

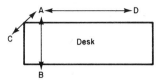

Fig. 3.2.   Three seating positions at a desk.

When position A-C is adopted there is six times more interaction than A-B and three times more than A-D. In non-medical studies, A-C is usually chosen when one person gives advice to another, A-D for a co-operative task, and A-B for a competitive task. The absence of a desk will normally reduce the perceived authority of the doctor unless he compensates in some other way, such as wearing a white coat.

This is not suggesting that there is a right and wrong position—it should vary with need—but as styles tend to be inflexible, appropriate variation probably occurs rarely.

5 DRESS

Doctors are expected to dress conservatively, and most do, but there is still a spectrum ranging from those General Practitioners who wear white coats, those wearing three-piece suits, casual suits, sports jackets, sweaters to open neck shirts and jeans. Clothes convey authority and a casually dressed Doctor is likely to be seen as a much less authoritarian figure than the one wearing the white coat. Group practices often seem to develop styles of dress. In one health centre that I know well, one partnership usually wear formal suits and the other sweaters and slacks. This difference in dress reflects many differences in character and attitude clearly perceived by the patients. Pursuing this theme briefly, it often appears that group practices develop a particular collection of behaviours and attitudes that are more than just the sum of the individual doctors. This may be for historical reasons and because of the common human desire to belong to a distinctive group. Whatever the reasons are, there is no doubt that different practices are recognized by patients as having particular styles.

6 INFORMATION GATHERING

The first phase of any consultation is usually concerned with the doctor gathering information. The opening statements will often dictate the path that the remainder of the consultation will follow. For example, "How is the diabetes today?" or "Hello, how is that back of yours?", give considerably less scope for response than "Hello, how can I help?" or the even more open "Hello, do sit down, now then . . ." or just "Good morning". Non-verbal behaviour is just as important and movements made by the doctor can greatly aid the establishment of rapport. This is particularly important in relation to eye contact. In a recent study, doctors, whose verbal behaviour was considered patient-centred, changed position significantly more frequently than those considered doctor-centred Byrne and Heath (1980).

It seems that most doctors develop stock openings consisting of both verbal and non-verbal behaviours, repeated time and again. When I first video-recorded myself consulting, I was chastened to see myself repeat virtually the same opening with all patients. This is a crucial phase in the consultation and awareness of our behaviour and some knowledge of the consequences is essential if we are to alter our behaviour to produce a more satisfactory result. For example, when the patient begins to talk, many doctors immediately go down a form of clinical check list. They have been trained that way and this technique quickly creates recognizable patterns that can be pigeon-holed and dealt with. This technique is characterized by a linked set of closed questions designed to exclude various possibilities while leading to a likely physical diagnosis. In general practice, it is also based on the fact that a working hypothesis has been made very early in the consultation. When using this method of gathering information, it is usually the presenting complaint that is fixed on, the implication being that the doctor is looking for answers that will enable him to solve that problem for the patient.

The consequence of this approach can be one of the greatest faults in modern general practice. This is the organization of vague symptoms into categories, then labelling these producing a disease that can be approached in the traditional medical manner. Having created a disease in this way, it becomes very difficult to unmake. This tendency is particularly obvious in the handling of the everyday emotional trauma all human beings experience. For example, unhappiness is a human condition, whereas "depression" is a disease that can be treated with anti-depressives. Medicalization is a name that has been given to this behaviour—and it deserves such an ugly word.

A different opening style is that of listening in the initial phase. The patient can be encouraged by the doctor's non-verbal behaviour, especially eye-contact, nodding the head and so on. Sensitively used, open ended questions can be especially helpful. This method has been likened to steering a canoe down the river, allowing it to flow freely just nudging it off the bank if need be.

Skilful exponents of this technique use silence as a means of allowing the patient to say what matters to him. Other skills include the use of the reflected question. For example, when the patient asks "Why do I get these headaches?" the doctor might reply "why do you think you get them?" This can reveal unexpected fears and beliefs crucial to the understanding of an illness. Simple open-ended questions can also help reveal much more of the patient's beliefs, feelings and effects of the illness (see Chapter 5, this volume). This more flexible and open style is not consistently taught in Medical School but demonstrations and discussions with trainees in the Oxford region has produced a great deal of enthusiasm, described by Pendleton and Tate (1980). Many doctors are only dimly aware that there are effective ways of gathering information other than the medical history taking model. There are encouraging signs that the next decade will see giant strides in this field. The booklet "Talking with Patients" produced by a Nuffield Working Party (1980) of very eminent medical men is a fine start.

There are a great many behavioural skills that can be involved in gathering information. Byrne and Long listed over fifty but two are worth considering briefly. The first is the skill of observing. When consultations are viewed directly or video-recorded, the fact that many doctors spend a lot of time writing and reading notes becomes apparent. Much non-verbal information is thus lost, missing important emotional clues. Rapport with a patient's feelings requires that the doctor must be aware of the nuances of gesture, eye-movement and body posture. In early studies of the consultation, the data were based solely on audio-tape recording and the whole subject of observation was omitted.

The other important skill that should be mentioned is that of the physical examination. This is an integral part of the information-gathering process and both its use and the manner in which it is carried out are likely to become stylized. An examination can be purely a way of seeking clinical information or it can be expanded into an impressive and powerful ritual. At no other time does the doctor exact such control over his patient and all doctors are aware of the therapeutic effect this can produce. For those doctors wishing to establish their authority over their patients the examination is most likely to be embellished and ritualized.

When studying consultations, it can be difficult to define when the phase of information-gathering ends. Often the doctor returns to questioning again and again until almost the end. Byrne and Long demonstrated that in many consultations when they observed this behaviour, it was because the doctor had failed to get to the root of why the patient had come to him. This can be clearly related to style. The doctor who only follows the path of the presenting remarks is very likely to miss any other reasons for attendance, producing a higher proportion of what has been termed dysfunctional consultations.

7 INFORMATION GIVING

Some of the skills that can be involved in the giving of information include explaining, sharing, advising, clarifying, dealing with questions and ideas and so on. It is the blend and quality which will dictate the overall style.

One definition of information is "that which reduces uncertainty" and, as discussed previously, maintaining uncertainty can be a method of maintaining influence. Doctors who habitually give little or cryptic information to their patients are consciously or unconsciously maintaining power over them. There is some evidence that the giving of information is related to patient satisfaction and this, in turn, is related to how well advice is complied with (see the chapter by Pendleton in this volume). This may mean that those doctors who habitually give advice but little information produce their therapeutic effect mainly by their authority.

There is considerable evidence on the relatively poor uptake of medical advice (see Chapter 1, this volume) and it is very probable that changes in style could improve this. The use of strategies, as indicated by the Health Belief Model, seems very likely to increase compliance, although there is always the niggling doubt that patients may be correct in the sifting of medical information and that, if doctors are to increase the uptake of medical advice, there is even more onus to ensure that the advice is sound.

When the subject of information giving to patients is discussed by doctors, the word "appropriate" crops up frequently. There is evidence from work by Pendleton and Bochner (1980) that many General Practitioners volunteer fewer explanations to lower social class patients believing that they require and understand less. This belief is reinforced by the fact that the lower social classes tend not to ask many direct questions but studies indicate that this may be due to different modes of expression. Working-class people want to know as much about their illnesses as middle-class people according to Cartwright (1964). When looking at a doctor's style of information-giving, the essential question to ask is on what grounds does he decide the appropriateness of his explanations? Is it that he gives advice to everybody in a similar way or does he try to modify it, depending on his conception of the patients' understanding and from what information does he derive this concept of the patient's understanding? It has been shown by Waitzkin and Stoekle (1972) that doctors under-estimate patients' knowledge of illness and those who most seriously under-estimate knowledge tend to communicate the least information. General Practitioners attribute knowledge to their patients, delve for information and motivation to learn about illness and this process of attribution involves complex decision-making rules which are probably not constant but vary according to the individual doctors. It may become a matter of style.

8 PRESCRIBING

In Chapter 9 (this volume), Ann Cartwright states that prescribing is usually related to communication and, in her study of ten General Practitioners, Norma Raynes (1980) found that prescribing was inversely associated with referring patients for evaluation or treatment. It appears that prescribing is a routine in General Practice—a relatively fixed part of any style. Prescribing patterns are little influenced by the presenting complaint except in relation to psychosocial problems and seem more often to be routines designed to terminate the consultation.

It is perhaps not surprising that this powerful behaviour has become a ritual. The therapeutic art of prescribing is still expected by most patients and their doctors, despite orchestrated campaigns designed to lessen these expectations. This is an area in which future training of General Practitioners must be concentrated to increase flexibility and appropriateness. The ultimate benefit to the national drug bill alone could be substantial.

9 TIME

When doctors discuss the reason for their behaviours, the commonest factor mentioned is one of time. The traditional authoritarian approach allows the doctor to control his use of time and structure his day. The average consultation in British general practice lasts about seven minutes and to maintain this average throughout a surgery of twenty or more patients requires some regulation on the part of the doctor. There is still considerable debate concerning the relative merits of the doctor-centred, clinically-oriented, fairly quick style of consulting as opposed to the much less structured, more time-consuming ideas and emotion-seeking style. Champions of the latter style argue that the extra time taken at one consultation discovering beliefs, anxieties and effects will be repaid by fewer consultations in the future. Studies are urgently needed to confirm or refute this belief for this debate is central to future training of doctors and proof is needed to convince die-hard medical educationalists that the adoption of a less structured, more time-consuming approach, is feasible.

10 IMPLICATIONS FOR TRAINING

Teaching doctors how to consult, as well as teaching them, clinical medicine has only recently become fashionable again, most obviously in the fields of psychiatry and general practice.

Stott and Davis (1979) have produced a very important aide memoire of the potential in each primary care consultation.

A	B
Management of presenting problems	Modification of help-seeking behaviours
C	D
Management of continuing problems	Opportunistic health position

This is a global view of the consultation and is a theoretical base from which to develop the full potential of any primary care consultation, it highlights some unique features of good general practice and is unashamedly patient centred. Attitudes harden and strong emotions are often generated when discussing areas B and D and it is this part of the framework which is noticeably weak in modern general practice and improving our skills in these two areas is the challenge to general practice training in the future.

Teaching behaviours and skills is time-consuming and difficult. Various techniques are employed, such as, direct observation by a third party sitting in, using a one-way mirror, recording by audiotape or videotape and the use of role play.

The use of audiotape and videotape have the advantage of being a permanent record and repeatable and are suitable for use in small groups. Videotape is far superior as a teaching tool because it includes the crucial non-verbal element and is more interesting, holding the group's attention much better than audiotape.

Having one's behaviour watched and dissected is very threatening to most of us, and, if done clumsily, feelings can be irrevocably hurt and the young doctor can retreat from such intrusions altogether. This puts great responsibility on those engaged in trying to teach behaviours. There should be certain ground rules and, in the Oxford region, we use the following. First, after watching any consultation, the discussion is centred solely on what is seen to be good or well done, the idea being to build on strengths not to criticize weaknesses. Secondly, there is a rule never to criticize without supporting as well. These rules are also used in one-to-one teaching. Particularly unsure and anxious doctors may initially find it best to watch their consultation alone before subjecting them to peer group scrutiny.

11 SUMMARY

Individual doctors vary in their style of consulting. His style is a unique blend of behaviours determined by his skills and his attitudes, and influenced by his personality, experience and education.

All doctors should be aware of the effects of their ways of behaving on their patients. Most importantly, we should learn that these behaviours are not immutable. We can all, with (a little) help (from our friends), learn new behaviours and skills, possibly bringing about changes in our attitudes. Future training of all doctors must be intimately concerned with the question of *style*.

REFERENCES

Bloor, M. (1978). On the routinised nature of work in people processing agencies. In *Relationships between Doctors and Patients* (A. Davis, ed.). Saxon House, London.

Byrne, P. S. and Heath, C. C. (1980). Practitioners' use of non-verbal behaviour in real consultations. *J. Roy. Coll. Gen. Pract.* **30**, 327–331.

Byrne, P. S. and Long, B. E. L. (1976). *Doctors Talking to Patients*. H.M.S.O., London.

Cartwright, A. (1964). *Human Relations and Hospital Care*. Routledge, London.

Fitton, F. and Acheson, H. W. (1979). *The Doctor Patient Relationship*. H.M.S.O., London.

Nuffield Working Party (1980). Talking with Patients, a teaching approach. Walton J. Sir. Nuffield Provincial Hospitals Trust.

Osmond, H. (1980). *New Eng. J. Med.* **302**, 555–558.

Pendleton, D. and Bochner, S. (1980). The communication of medical information in general practice consultations as a function of patients' social class. *Soc. Sci. Med.* **14A**, 669–673.

Pendleton, D. and Tate, P. (submitted for publication). The role of the psychologist in primary care: the non-clinical alternative. Paper presented at the Annual Conference of the British Psychological Society, Aberdeen, 1980.

Pietroni, P. (1976). Non-verbal communication in the general practice surgery. In *Language and Communication in General Practice* (B. Tanner, ed.). Hodder and Stoughton, London.

Raynes, N. V. (1980). *J. Roy. Coll. Gen. Pract.* **30**, 166–171.

Stott, N. C. H. and Davis, R. H. (1979). The exceptional potential in each primary care consultation. *J. Roy. Coll. Gen. Pract.* **29**, 201–205.

Waitzkin, H. and Stoeckle, J. D. (1972). The communication of information about illness. *Adv. Psychosom. Med.* **8**, 180–215.

Part II
Psychological Perspectives on the Consultation

4 Patients' Understanding and Recall in Clinical Communication failure

Philip Ley

1 A SIMPLE PARTIAL MODEL OF FAILURES OF CLINICAL COMMUNICATION

Two enduring important problems in the field of health care are that of presenting information about their illness to patients in such a way that they feel that they have been satisfactorily informed; and that of patients' non-compliance with advice from health professionals. Both of these became recognized as major problems during the 1960s. The problem of hospital patients' dissatisfaction with communications received attention not only from researchers but also from official bodies, e.g. Central Health Services Council, D.H.S.S. (1963). Research into this problem was reported by, amongst others, McGhee (1961), Cartwright (1964), Hugh-Jones *et al.* (1964), Spelman *et al.* (1966), Houghton (1968) and Raphael (1969). This research suggested that (a) dissatisfaction with communications was common; (b) dissatisfaction rates for communications were probably higher than for other areas of hospital stay; and (c) dissatisfaction rates were *not* lowered when clinicians were aware of the problem and made conscious attempts to overcome it (Ley 1972a, 1976). Despite the attention this problem received there is no evidence from more recent surveys to suggest that it has been solved or even that it has lessened in magnitude. Indeed studies with groups of general practice patients (Kincey *et al.* 1975; Ley, 1980a); studies of psychiatric patients (Raphael and Peers, 1972; Carstairs, 1970) and surveys conducted in the U.S.A. suggest that this problem is not confined merely to British hospital in-patients. Table 4.1, which is based on the reviews of Ley (1977) and Ley (1980b), summarizes this evidence.

Table 4.1. Dissatisfaction with communications amongst different types of patient.

Type of patient		% dissatisfied Median	Range
(a)	British hospital in-patients		
	1960–1970	35	11–65
	1971–1979	53	18–65
(b)	British general-practice patients	35	21–51
(c)	British psychiatric in-patients	39	31–54
(d)	Various U.S.A. patient groups	36	8–51

Whether the lack of improvement from the 1960s to the 1970s can be interpreted simply as the result of doctors remaining poor communicators in this area, or whether it is due to the effects of improved communication by health care personnel being obscured by rising patient expectations of what they should be told cannot be decided on the basis of available data. Objective records of the adequacy of communications for the two periods are lacking.

The problem of patients' non-compliance with advice is an important one in that it would appear that on average there is about one chance in two that a patient will not follow advice. Relevant evidence from the reviews of Ley (1977), Food and Drug Administration (1979) and Barofsky (1980) is summarized in Table 4.2.

Table 4.2. Frequency with which patients fail to follow advice about medication.

Type of medication	Ley (1972c)	Food and Drug Administration (1979)	Barofsky (1980)
Antibiotics	39	42	43
Psychiatric	39	42	42
Anti-hypertensive	—	43	61
Anti-tuberculosis	39	42	43
Other medication	48	54	46
Range of percents not complying	8–92	11–95	6–83

Before discussing the problem further it should, perhaps be stated that it cannot of course be assumed that patients should necessarily follow the advice they are given. Indeed attempts to increase compliance are fraught with ethical problems. Most of these would be overcome if compliance–induction attempts always involved the following steps:

(1) presentation to the patient of information on the effectiveness (and risks) of various possible treatments;

(2) a decision by the patient to try one or none of the treatments;

(3) if the patient decides to pursue a given treatment, compliance–induction is allowable provided that:

(4) there are regular opportunities for the patient to withdraw from treatment.

It is probable that this sequence of steps is not always followed when patients are given advice.

Interestingly enough it would seem from correlational studies that patients who feel satisfied with the communications aspect of consultations are more likely to follow advice. These investigations are summarized in Table 4.3.

Table 4.3. Correlations between satisfaction with communications and reported compliance amongst general practice patients in the U.K.

Investigation		Correlation	P
Kincey *et al.* 1975		Chi-square	<0.05
Ley *et al.* (1976b)	a.	+0·23	<0·05
	b.	+0·67	<0·001
Ley (1980b)		+0·19	n.s.

One other team of investigators has reported similar findings. In their study of paediatric out-patients Korsch and her collaborators found a strong correlation between satisfaction with the consultation and compliance with advice (Francis *et al.* 1969). Satisfaction with the consultation is obviously not necessarily the same as satisfaction with communications but it is plausible to suppose that these variables will correlate significantly with one another. For example Korsch *et al.* (1968) found that of patients who saw their doctor as a good communicator 86% were satisfied with the consultation as a whole, as opposed to only 25% who saw him as a bad communicator.

It would be expected that a number of variables would affect patients' levels of satisfaction with communications. These include the amount and content of the message; the way in which the clinician delivers it; the relationship between patient and clinician; contextual factors, e.g. the physical setting; and the individual characteristics of the patient. Of these the amount and content of what is said to patients is of overwhelming importance. It remains true that for whatever reasons many clinicians still fail to give patients information in areas where they would like it. This has been found in studies which have used patients' report of whether they had been told about an area, and in studies where an objective record of the consultation has been made (Ley, 1980a). If the clinician has not given the patient information it is not surprising that patients' levels of dissatisfaction are high. However, what makes this an interesting problem is that, as mentioned above, investigations of satisfaction rates in conditions where the clinicians have made conscious efforts to communicate show them to be no higher (Hugh-Jones *et al.*, 1964; Spelman *et al.*, 1966; Houghton, 1968).

Two factors seem particularly important in producing failures even when the clinician is trying. These are (a) the extent to which the patient understands the information presented and (b) the extent to which the patient remembers the message. These would seem to be necessary albeit not sufficient conditions for both patients' satisfaction with communications and their compliance with advice (Ley and Spelman, 1967). Further, as failures of understanding and memory are common, it should be empirically true that they will be major factors in both dissatisfaction and non-compliance.

Evidence of patients' failures to understand what they have been told by health-care personnel comes from four main sources. These are: patients' reports of not understanding; general medical knowledge tests; direct tests of understanding of what has been said; readability measurement of information given to patients. Investigations using these methods all suggest that patients frequently fail to understand what they are told.

Ley (1980b) reviewed three investigations of general practice patients. The percentage of patients claiming not to have understood the information on various aspects of their condition ranged from 7 to 47 for diagnosis; 17–47 for aetiology; 14–43 for treatment; and 13–53 for prognosis. This method of assessment would be expected to overestimate patients' understanding as replies are likely to be influenced by demand characteristics (for example, patients might assume that the information might get back to their doctors), and because patients might wrongly think that they have understood.

The use of general medical knowledge tests is a very indirect method of assessing the likelihood that patients would understand information they are given. At best the use of this technique can unearth common misconceptions, and sometimes it has done this. For example, Spelman and Ley (1966) found that laypersons commonly thought that the prognosis for lung cancer is good, and Boyle (1970) found that surprisingly large percentages of his sample did not know the approximate location of major organs. If common misconceptions exist, then it is likely that there will be many failures of comprehension of information related to these misconceptions.

Direct tests of patients' understanding of what they have been told have often assessed patients' understanding of prescription instructions. A number of such studies have been reviewed by Ley (1980a) who concluded that the percentage of patients who do not properly understand their prescription instructions ranges from 35 to 87%.

The final method of assessing understanding is the use of readability formulae. These formulae enable one to estimate the percentage of the population who will understand written materials. A number of investigations have applied these to written information about health related topics (Ley *et al.*, 1973; Ley, 1974; Pyrczak and Roth, 1976; French *et al.*, 1978; Liguori, 1978; Department of Health, Education and Welfare, 1979). The results of these studies are summarized in Table 4.4.

Table 4.4. Understandability of health related written information as assessed by readability formulae.

Material	Number of leaflets likely to be understood by stated % of population			
	25% or less	26–40%	41–74%	75% or more
X-ray leaflets (Ley *et al.*, 1972)	—	2	—	3
Dental leaflets (Ley, 1974)	1	1	—	3
Non prescription drug leaflets (Pyrczak and Roth, 1976)	6	3	—	1
Prescription drug leaflets (Liguori, 1978)	—	2	—	2
Opticians leaflets (French *et al.*, 1978)	7	20	9	2
Pamphlets about cancer (Dept of Health Education and Welfare, 1979)	6	2	—	—
All of the above	20	30	9	11

It can be seen that over 70% of these written communications would be understood by less than half of the population.

This brief review of the evidence shows conclusively that failures of understanding are likely to occur frequently. This raises the interesting problem of why clinicians should continue to communicate so poorly. The most likely answer is that patients, because of diffidence, do not ask questions when they do not understand (Cartwright, 1964; Ley and Spelman, 1967; Roter, 1977). This deprives the clinician of the feedback necessary for the improved communication.

As well as the difficulties caused by patients' failures to understand what they are told, there are the difficulties arising from patients' failures to remember the information given to them (Ley and Spelman, 1965, 1967; Joyce et al., 1969; Ley et al., 1973; Ley et al., 1976b; Anderson et al., 1979). The results of these investigations are summarized in Table 4.5.

Table 4.5. Patie nts forgetting of information given them by their doctors.

Investigation		Patients	% forgotten
Ley and Spelman (1965)		Medical out-patients	37
Ley and Spelman (1967)	(a)	Medical out-patients	39
	(b)	Medical out-patients	41
Joyce et al. (1969)	(a)	Rheumatological out-patients	52
	(b)	Rheumatological out-patients	54
Ley, et al. (1973)		General practice	50
Ley et al. (1976b)		General practice	44
Anderson et al. (1979)		Rheumatological out-patients	61

Forgetting is associated with the amount of information presented; the nature of the material; the patient's age, level of anxiety and medical knowledge (Ley, 1979b

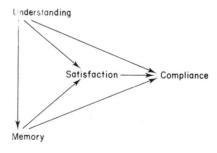

Fig. 4.1. Relationships between understanding, memory satisfaction and compliance.

These findings and those reviewed earlier led to the construction of the plausible simple model shown in Fig. 4.1.

Whether patients will comply with advice will depend in part on whether they have understood and remembered what they have been told, and on their level of satisfaction with communications. In turn satisfaction with communications will be partly dependent on memory and understanding. Finally understanding should affect the probability of information being recalled.

This simple model leads to the predictions that:

(1) increases in understanding will lead to increases in satisfaction and compliance;

(2) increases in memory will lead to increases in satisfaction and compliance;

(3) increases in satisfaction will lead to increases in compliance.

It is hardly necessary to emphasize that the model should not be considered as a complete account of the problem. The claim is rather that comprehension and memory account for a substantial part of the variance in both dissatisfaction and compliance and that manipulation of these variables will lead to increased control. Consideration of other variables affecting compliance and satisfaction will be deferred until after a review of the evidence related to this simple model.

2 THE ADEQUACY OF THE MODEL

The first set of predictions consists of the predictions:

(1) that increased understanding will lead to increased memory;

(2) that increased understanding (and if the first prediction is correct, increased memory) will lead to increased satisfaction with communications;

(3) that increased understanding (and memory) will lead to increased compliance.

Ley and his co-workers have conducted a number of experiments to see whether increased understanding leads to increased recall of medical information. These experiments have compared recall of information written to produce varying levels of readability as measured by the Flesch Formula (Flesch, 1948). The control material has always been material in ordinary clinical use, and the experimental material has consisted of the same information written in shorter words and shorter sentences (simplification). The results of these experiments are summarized in Table 4.6, where it will be seen that overall the evidence supports the hypothesis.

The second hypothesis, that increased comprehension and memory will lead to increased satisfaction with communications gains some support from both correlational and experimental evidence. The correlational evidence is drawn from four studies of general practice patients and one study of surgical

Table 4.6. Effects of increasing understanding by simplification on recall of medical
information.

Investigation	Material		Mean % increase in recall as a result of simplification	P
Ley *et al.* (1972)	X-ray	1.	−6	n.s.
	information	2.	+34	<0·01
Bradshaw *et al.* (1975)	Dietary	1.	+29	n.s.
	information	2.	+72	<0·05
		3.	+48	<0·01
Ley *et al.* (1979)	Menopause information		+21	<0·05

Table 4.7. Correlations between reported comprehension and reported satisfaction
with communications.

Investigation	Patients		Correlation	P
Kincey *et al.* (1975)	General practice		Chi-square	<0·05
Ley *et al.* (1976a)	a.	General practice	+0·69	<0·001
	b.	General practice	+0·64	<0·001
Ley (1980b)	a.	General practice	+0·68	<0·001
	b.	Surgical	+0·45	<0·001

inpatients. The correlations found are given in Table 4.7.

The results of these investigations are consistent in showing reasonably high correlations between *reported* understanding and satisfaction with communications.

Attempts to obtain experimental evidence to support the hypothesis have been reported by Ley *et al.* (1976a), and Ley (1980b). The first of these investigations compared levels of post-discharge satisfaction with the communications aspect of hospital stay amongst medical ward patients. These patients had been assigned randomly to the usual hospital procedure (control); the experimental procedure, in which a houseman paid the patient an extra visit to ensure that the patient had understood the information presented; or to a placebo condition, in which a houseman paid extra visits, but talked about such topics as privacy, comfort and the like. (Full details are given in the paper by Ley *et al.*, 1976a.) It was found that the patients in the experimental group were significantly more likely to be satisfied with communications.

The second experiment involved surgical in-patients and had essentially the same design as the experiment with medical ward patients. This time there were no significant differences between groups. The results of these two experiments are shown in Table 4.8.

Table 4.8. Effects of attempts to increase understanding on satisfaction with communications.

Group	% satisfied: Medical patients	Surgical patients
Control	52	75
Placebo	41	84
Experimental	80	72
	($P<0·05$)	(n.s.)

The reasons for these different results are not immediately apparent, but it is noticeable that the surgical patients in the control and placebo groups had significantly higher levels of satisfaction than their medical counterparts. It is therefore possible that the failure to obtain the desired result was due to a ceiling effect. It is also worth recalling that amongst the surgical patients there was a significant correlation between reported understanding and satisfaction (see Table 4.7).

Some apparently negative evidence is also reported by Hulka (1979). This investigator and her co-workers reported very low correlation between a communication score (the amount a patient knows as a ratio of what the clinician wants him to know) and a satisfaction score. The satisfaction score is a compound score derived from attitude measures whose objects are (a) the physician's competence; (b) the personal qualities of the physician; and (c) the cost and convenience of care. This is clearly not a direct test of the hypothesis about understanding and satisfaction with communications, but it diminishes the temptation to generalize from satisfaction with communications to other measures of satisfaction. The third prediction is that increased understanding/memory will lead to increased compliance. Once more some correlational evidence is available which is summarized in Table 4.9.

Table 4.9. Correlations between reported comprehension and reported compliance amongst general practice patients.

Investigation	Correlation	P
Kincey *et al.* (1975)	Chi-square	<0·10
Ley *et al.* (1976b)	a. +0·31	<0·01
	b. +0·57	<0·01
Ley (1980b)	+0·20	<0·05

In addition to this correlational evidence, there is some relevant experimental evidence. One such experiment was conducted by Ley *et al.* (1975). The subjects were a group of 80 depressed and 80 anxious psychiatric outpatients. These patients within each group were randomly assigned to one of four conditions. These were the usual hospital procedure (no leaflet about medication), and three experimental conditions: difficult leaflet, moderate leaflet and easy leaflet. The leaflets gave brief information about the medication, and varied in difficulty as assessed by the Flesch Formula. The dependent variable was a medication error score which was derived by expressing the difference between tablets prescribed and tablets taken, as a percentage of tablets prescribed. The results were the same for both groups of patients, and showed that the difficult leaflet was ineffective in reducing medication errors but that the moderate and easy leaflets led to significant reductions in such errors, the easy leaflet being significantly better than the moderate one in this respect. The results are summarized in Table 4.10.

However, it is clear from the review of Morris and Halperin (1979) that the

Table 4.10. Effects of leaflets of varying difficulty on medication errors made by patients.

Leaflet condition	Mean medication error (%)	
	Anxious patients	Depressed patients
None	15	16
Difficult	15	15
Moderate	8	8
Easy	6	3

provision of written information does not always increase compliance. These authors reviewed eighteen investigations into the effects of such information on compliance and concluded that in only twelve of the studies was compliance increased. However, the present hypothesis is that increased comprehension will lead to increased compliance, and in only five of the investigations reviewed by Morris and Halperin was it demonstrated that there had been a significant gain in patients' understanding as a result of the provision of a leaflet. (Madden, 1973; Sackett *et al.*, 1975; McKenney *et al.*, 1973; MacDonald *et al.*, 1977; Boyd *et al.*, 1974.) In only one of these (Sackett *et al.*, 1975) was increased knowledge not associated with increased compliance.

Finally, Hulka (1979) reports a correlation between her communication score and compliance amongst patients with heart failure but not amongst those with diabetes.

Overall these results are generally in favour of the hypothesis concerning comprehension. Increased comprehension appears to lead to increased recall of information presented by doctors, to increased satisfaction with communications, and to increased compliance. However, there are sufficient negative findings in this last area to demand refinement of the hypothesis. A similar mixture of positive and negative findings emerges from investigations of the effects of increasing memory on compliance.

Several methods have been evolved for presenting information to patients in such a way as to enhance the probability of their recalling it. These include simplification (Ley *et al.*, 1972; Bradshaw *et al.*, 1975); explicit categorization (Ley *et al.*, 1973); repetition (Kupst *et al.*, 1975; Ley, 1979b); and use of specific rather than general advice statements (Bradshaw *et al.*, 1975). In addition, the content of what is recalled can be influenced by the manipulation of primacy and importance effects (Ley, 1972b). Finally, package mixtures of these techniques can sometimes lead to increased recall (Ley *et al.*, 1976b) but not always (Ley *et al.*, 1979). The results of experiments on the effects of simplification in increasing recall of medical information have already been presented in Table 4.6. A summary of the results of experiments on the other memory enhancing techniques is given in Table 4.11.

Apart from the investigation of the effects of increased understanding/ memory on the accuracy of medicine-taking which has already been described, the experiments of Ley and his co-workers on the effects of increased memory on compliance have involved packages of memory—enhancing techniques. Ley (1978) reported the results of three experiments to assess the effects of increasing the memorability of written information concerning obesity and dieting on weight loss amongst obese females. These women received all their information in written form. One version was moderately easy as assessed by the Flesch Formula, the other, the experimental version, was simplified and contained explicit categorization and repetition. Despite a very impressive

Table 4.11. Effects of explicit categorization, repetition use of specific advice statements, and combinations of these on recall of medical information.

Investigations	Subjects		% improvement in recall	P
1. *Explicit categorization*				
Ley *et al*. (1973	general practice patients		+24%	<0·01
Ley (1979b)	7 analogue studies		+31%	<0·01
2. *Repetition*				
Kupst *et al*. (1975)	parents of children		+20%	<0·01
Ley (1979b)	6 analogue studies		+31%	<0·01
3. *Use of specific advice statements*				
Bradshaw *et al*. (1975)	obese women	a.	+350%	<0·001
		b.	+158%	<0·001
		c.	+219%	<0·001
4. *Mixtures of techniques*				
Ley *et al*. (1976).	general practice patients		+27%	<0·001
Ley *et al*. (1979b)	general practice patients		−6%	n.s.

result in the first experiment two further attempts to repeat the findings met with no success. The results are summarized in Table 4.12.

Table 4.12. Effects of increased comprehension and memory on weight loss.

Booklet	Mean weight loss in lb at 8 weeks		
	Exp. 1	Exp. 2	Exp. 3
Standard	7·7	8·3	10·3
Increased comprehensibility and memorability	12·3	7·5	9·9
(P)	(<0·01)	(n.s.)	(n.s.)

As the subjects were recruited in the same way from the same population this set of results is hard to explain. Possible explanations are discussed by Ley *et al*. (1980), but whatever the reasons it is clear that there is a great deal of variance not explained by this simple model.

The last prediction from this model is that satisfaction with communications should be related to compliance. Correlational evidence has already been presented in Table 4.3, but there seems to be a dearth of experimental evidence. A possibly relevant investigation is that of Roter (1979). Roter did not deliberately attempt to manipulate satisfaction with communications, rather she tried to increase question-asking during the consultations by patients.

This attempt was successful but led to more anger and anxiety amongst both patients and clinicians, and, by inference, less satisfaction. Despite this the manipulation led to greater compliance in appointment keeping. Indeed in the experimental groups there was a positive correlation between negative affect experienced and compliance, while in the control group this correlation was negative. (Of course it is not necessarily true that experiencing anger and anxiety reduced satisfaction with communications or with the consultation overall.)

3 DISCUSSION

Despite the mixed findings reviewed above it is clear that comprehension and memory are important factors in both patients' satisfaction and their compliance with advice. The effects of these variables appear to range from their being apparently ineffective to their accounting for a substantial part of the variance in dissatisfaction and non-compliance. Possible reasons for these disparaties in effectiveness include (a) difficulties arising from the rather loose definition of these concepts, and (b) the existence of other powerful variables in compliance which can attenuate the effects of increased comprehension and memory.

Although satisfaction with communications is relatively easily assessed either generally or in relation to specific areas of medical information, e.g. diagnosis, prognosis, aetiology, treatment, there appear to be no investigations of the relationships of these specific components to overall satisfaction with communications. Nor is the relationship of satisfaction with communications to satisfaction with other aspects of the consultation known. It is clearly possible that satisfaction with communications exerts whatever effects it has on compliance via its effect on general satisfaction with the encounters with the clinician.

More analytic definitions of comprehension and compliance will also be needed in future research. To date in investigations of medication compliance the term comprehension has been variously used to denote:

(1) understanding of the illness;

(2) understanding the rationale of treatment;

(3) understanding the mechanics of treatment, e.g. when to take a pill, how to take it, how many pills to take.

Non-compliance has also had a variety of meanings attributed to it. These have included:

(1) not taking the medicine at all;

(2) taking the medicine wrongly;

(3) taking medicines other than those prescribed (Hulka, 1979).

Further complications can arise from consideration of the characteristics of the non-complying patient. Ley (1979a) has suggested that such patients can be crudely classified along two dimensions according to whether their non-compliance is intentional or unintentional, and according to whether or not they have adequate or inadequate information. Intentional non-compliers will be those who have decided not to follow the treatment advice either because of enduring attitudinal predispositions, e.g. that medication is an undesirable treatment; or because in a particular instance they consider that the benefits of treatment are outweighed by its risks and disadvantages. Within this group it is only those who have an inadequate amount of information who are likely to be affected by the provision of fuller further information.

The unintentional non-complier is probably making scheduling errors. Some of these patients will be perfectly well aware of when they should take their medicines but due to lapses of memory or attention not take their medicines at the right times, while others will not have correct knowledge about when to take the medicines. They will wrongly think that they are taking it properly. This last group would also be likely to be affected by the provision of information. It can be seen that the success of any attempt to increase comprehension and memory would be strongly influenced by the relative proportions of non-compliers falling into these different groups. For example, percentages of patients not adequately informed of the details of treatment range from approximately 17% (Hulka, 1979) to 87% (Mazullo et al., 1974). An attempt to increase compliance by increasing comprehension would be much more likely to succeed in the second than in the first case. Thus it can be seen that the effectiveness of providing information will depend on the interaction of (a) the nature of the information, (b) the type of non-compliance, and (c) the type of non-complier.

Indeed it is theoretically possible that the provision of certain sorts of information could increase non-compliance. (Once more it should be emphasized that this might not necessarily be a bad thing.) It is interesting to note that in the investigation of Sackett et al. (1975), patients exposed to mastery learning were slightly less likely to be compliant (50% as opposed to 44%). It is also widely suspected by clinicians that the provision of information about the risks of investigative procedures and treatments would reduce compliance with advice to undertake those treatments. There is not a great deal of evidence available on this topic, but that reviewed by Ley (1980a) suggests that the provision of such information leads to no noticeable reduction in compliance with advice. Thus, for example, in the investigations of the effects of informing patients about the side-effects of medications there is no support for the contention that the provision of such information increases either non-compliance or the probability of experiencing side-effects (Myers and Calvert, 1973, 1976, 1978; Newcomer and Anderson, 1974; Elklund and Wessling, 1976; Paulson *et al.*, 1976; Suveges, 1977; Weibert, 1977).

This digression has raised the question of the role of factors other than comprehension, memory and satisfaction in compliance. Ley (1979) reviewing the literature concluded that to date the main proven determinants of compliance with medical advice were those shown in Fig. 4.2.

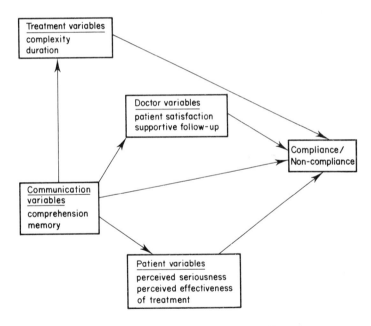

Fig. 4.2.   Variables affecting non-compliance.

Complexity and duration of treatment have the expected effects on non-compliance and patient satisfaction variables have been discussed already. Yet another piece of doctor behaviour which seems to exert a strong effect is the provision of supportive follow-up and while in general the search for individual difference correlates of compliance has been unsuccessful, research on the Health Belief Model variables supports the view that perceived vulnerability to, perceived seriousness of the illness affect compliance as does the perceived efficacy of treatment.

Increases in comprehension and memory would be expected to affect non-compliance directly, and indirectly by their effects on patients' satisfaction and patients' perceptions of their vulnerability, the seriousness of the illness, and the efficacy of treatment, and by reducing errors caused by the complexity of the treatment regimen. However, the overall outcome of increases in memory and comprehension would depend on the magnitude of the effects exerted by the other variables shown in Fig. 4.2.

It should be emphasized that these variables are those which research to date has established as having effects on compliance. While it is true that a number of other possible variables have proved not to be correlated with compliance (for a full list see the annotated bibliography and summaries in Haynes *et al.*, 1979), several of the message and other variables studied by social psychologists interested in attitude change seem likely to be of value (Ley and Spelman 1967; Ley *et al.*, 1974; Skilbeck *et al.*, 1977; Ley 1980b, 1980c).

Finally brief mention should be made of the possible ways of increasing the feedback that the clinician receives from the patient. Theoretically such increased feedback should improve the clinician's communicative performance. A technique worthy of further investigation in this respect is the patient-activation technique described by Roter (1977). This consisted of a pre-consultation interview with a health educator who used a check list to assess what information the patient would like and then, if necessary, trained and rehearsed the patient in how to ask for this information.

Even more novel is the idea proposed by Fischbach *et al.* (1979), that patients should be made co-authors of their case notes. Both of these techniques should significantly increase the amount of feedback to clinicians.

REFERENCES

Anderson, J. L., Dodman, S., Kopelman, M. and Fleming, A. (1979). Patient information recall in a rheumatology clinic. *Rheumatol. Rehabil.* **18**, 18–22.

Barofsky, I. (1980). *The Chronic Psychiatric Patient in the Community*. Plenum Press, New York.

Boyd, J. R., Covington, T. R., Stanaszek, W. F. and Coussons, R. T. (1974). Drug defaulting, part II: analysis of non-compliance patterns. *Am. J. Hosp. Pharm.* **31**, 485–491.

Boyle, C. M. (1970). Differences between doctors' and patients' interpretations of some common medical terms. *Br. Med. J.* **2**, 286–289.

Bradshaw, P. W., Ley, P., Kincey, J. A. and Bradshaw, J. (1975). Recall of medical advice: comprehensibility and specificity. *Br. J. Soc. Clin. Psychol.* **14**, 55–62.

Carstairs, V. (1970). *Channels of Communication*. Scottish Home and Health Depart-

ment, Edinburgh.
Cartwright, A. (1964). *Human Relations and Hospital Care*. Routledge and Kegan Paul, London.
Department of Health and Social Security (1963). *Communications between Doctors, Nurses and Patients*. H.M.S.O., London.
Department of Health, Education & Welfare (1979). Readability testing in cancer communications. Warlington D.C. DHEW Publications No. (NIH) 79–1689.
Eklund, L. H. and Wessling, A. (1976). Evaluation of package enclosures for drug packages. *Lakaridningen* 73, 2319–2320.
Fischbach, R. L., Bayog, A. S., Needle, A. and Delbanco, T. L. (1980). The patient and practitioner as co-authors of the medical record. *Pat. Counsell. Health Educ.* 2, 1–5.
Flesch, R. (1948). A new readability yardstick. *J. Appl. Psychol.* 32, 221–233.
Food and Drug Administration (1979). Prescription drug products: patient labelling requirements. *Federal Register* 44, 40016–40041.
Francis, V., Korsch, B. M. and Morris M. J. (1969). Gaps in doctor–patient communication: patients response to medical advice. *New Engl. J. Med.* 280, 535–540.
French, C., Mellor, M. and Parry, L. (1978). Patients' views of the ophthalmic optician. *Ophthalmic optician*, 28th October, 784–786.
Haynes, R. B., Taylor, D. W. and Sackett, D. L. (1979). *Compliance in Health Care*. John Hopkins University Press, Baltimore.
Houghton, M. (1968). Problems in hospital communication. In *Problems and Progress in Medical Care* (G. MacLachlan, (ed.). Nuffield Provincial Hospitals Trust, London.
Hugh-Jones, P. Tanser, A. F. and Whitby, C. (1964). Patients' view of admission to a London Teaching Hospital. *Br. Med. J.* 2, 660–664.
Hulka, B. S. (1979). Patient–clinician interaction and compliance. In *Compliance in Health Care* (R. B. Haynes, D. W. Taylor and D. L. Sackett, eds). John Hopkins University Press, Baltimore.
Joyce, C. R. B., Caple, G., Mason, M., Reynolds, E. and Matthews, J. A. (1969). Quantitative study of doctor–patient communication. *Quart. J. Med.* 38, 183–194.
Kincey, J. A., Bradshaw, P. W. and Ley, P. (1975). Patients satisfaction and reported acceptance of advice in general practice. *J. Roy. Coll. Gen. Pract.* 25, 558–566.
Korsch, B. M., Gozzi, E. K. and Francis, V. (1968). Gaps in doctor–patient communication: doctor–patient interaction and patient satisfaction. *Pediatrics* 42, 855–871.
Kupst, M. J., Dresser, K., Schulman, J. L. and Paul, M. H. (1975). Evaluation of methods to improve communication in the physician patient relationship. *Am. J. Orthopsychiat.* 45, 420–429.
Ley, P. (1972a). Complaints by hospital staff and patients: a review of the literature. *Bull. Br. Psychol. Soc.* 25, 115–120.
Ley, P. (1972b). Primacy, rated importance and the recall of medical information. *J. Health Soc. Behav.* 13, 311–317.
Ley, P. (1974). Communication in the clinical setting. *Br. J. Orthodont.* 1, 173–177.
Ley, P. (1976). Towards better doctor–patient communication: contributions from social and experimental psychology. In *Communication between Doctors and Patients* A. E. Bennett, (ed.). Nuffield Provincial Hospitals Trust, London.
Ley, P. (1977). Psychological studies of doctor–patient communication. In *Contributions to Medical Psychology, Vol. 1*. (S. Rachman, ed.). Pergamon Press, Oxford.

Ley, P. (1978). Psychological and behavioural factors in weight loss. In *Recent Advances in Obesity Research, Vol. 2*. (G. A. Bray, ed.). Newman Publishing, London.

Ley, P. (1979a). The psychology of compliance. In *Research in Psychology and Medicine, Vol. 2*. (D. J. Oborne, M. M. Gruneberg and J. R. Eiser, eds). Academic Press, London.

Ley, P. (1979b). Memory for medical information. *Br. J. Soc. Clin. Psychol.* **18**, 245–256.

Ley, P. (1980a). Giving information to patients. In *Social Psychology and Behavioural Medicine* (J. R. Eiser, ed.). Wiley, London.

Ley, P. (1980b). *Communication Variables in Health Education*. Health Education Council Monographs, London.

Ley, P. (1980c). The psychology of obesity. In *Contributions to medical psychology, 2* (S. Rachman, ed.). Oxford: Pergamon Press.

Ley P. and Spelman, M. S. (1965). Communications in an out-patient setting. *British Journal of Social and Clinical Psychology*, **4**, 114–116.

Ley, P. and Spelman, M. S. (1967). *Communicating with the Patient*. Staples Press, London.

Ley, P., Goldman, M., Bradshaw, P. W., Kincey, J. A. and Walker, C. (1972). The comprehensibility of some x-ray leaflets. *J. Inst. Health Educ.* **10**, 47–53.

Ley, P., Bradshaw, P. W., Eaves, D. and Walker, C. M. (1973). A method for increasing patients recall of information presented by doctors. *Psychol. Med.* **3**, 217–2230.

Ley, P., Jain, V. K. and Skilbeck, C. E. (1975). A method for decreasing patients medication errors. *Psychol. Med.* **6**, 599–601.

Ley, P., Bradshaw, P. W., Kincey, J. A. and Atherton, S. T. (1976a). Increasing patients' satisfaction with communications. *Br. J. Soc. Clin. Psychol.* **15**, 403–413.

Ley, P., Whitworth, M. A., Skilbeck, C. E., Woodward, R., Pinsent, R. J. F. H., Pike, L. A., Clarkson, M. E. and Clark, P. B. (1976b). Improving doctor–patient communications in general practice. *J. Roy. Coll. Gen. Pract.* **26**, 720–724.

Ley, P., Pike, L. A. Whitworth, M. A. and Woodward, R. (1979). Effects of source, context of communication, and difficulty level on the success of health educational communications. *Health Educ. J.* **38**, 47–52.

Ley, P., Kincey, J. A., Whitworth, M. A. *et al.* (1980). Problems in the instigation and short term maintenance of weight loss: results of fourteen experiments. Appendix to Ley, P. *Communication Variables in Health Education*. Health Education Council Monographs, London.

Liguori, S. (1978). A quantitative assessment of the readability of PPIs. *Drug Intell. Clin. Pharm.* **12**, 712–716.

MacDonald, E. T., MacDonald, J. B. and Phoenix, M. (1977). Improving drug compliance after hospital discharge. *Br. Med. J.* **2**, 618–621.

McGhee, A. (1961). *The Patients Attitude to Nursing Care*. Livingstone, Edinburgh.

McKenney, J. M., Slining, J. M. and Henderson, H. R. (1973). The effect of clinical pharmacy services on patients with essential hypertension. *Circulation* **48**, 1104–1111.

Madden, E. E. (1973). Evaluation of out-patient pharmacy counselling. *J. Am. Pharmaceut. Assoc.* **13**, 437–443.

Mazzullo, J. M., Cohn, K., Lasagne, L. and Griner, P. F. (1974). Variations in interpretation of presciption instructions. *J. Amer. Med. Assoc.*, **227**, 929–931.

Morris, L. A. and Halperin, J. (1979). Effects of written drug information on patient knowledge and compliance: a literature review. *Am. J. Pub. Health* **69**, 47–52.

Myers, E. D. and Calvert, E. J. (1973). Effects of forewarning on the occurrence of side-effects and discontinuance of medication in patients on amitryptiline. *Br. J. Psychiat* **122**, 461–464.

Myers, E. D. and Calvert, E. J. (1976). Effect of forewarning on the occurrence of side-effects and discontinuance of medication in patients on dothiepen. *J. Int. Med. Res.* **4**, 237–240.

Myers, E. D. and Calvert, E. J. (1978). Knowledge of side effects and perseverance with medication. *Br. J. Psychiat* **132**, 526–527.

Newcomer, D. R. and Anderson, R. W. (1974). Effectiveness of a combined drug self administration and patient teaching program. *Drug Intell. Clin. Pharm.* **8**, 374–381.

Paulson, P. T., Bauch, R., Paulson, M. L. and Zilz, D. A. (1976). Medication data sheets—an aid to patient education. *Drug Intell. Clin. Pharm.* **10**, 448–453.

Pyrczak, R. and Roth, D. H. (1976). The readability of directions on non-prescription drugs. *J. Am. Pharmaceut. Assoc.* **16**, 242–242, 267.

Raphael, W. (1969). *Patients and their Hospitals*. King Edward's Fund, London.

Raphael, W. and Peers, V. (1972). *Psychiatric Patients View their Hospitals*. King Edward's Fund, London.

Roter, D. (1977). Patient participation in the patient–provider interaction. *Health Educ. Mon.* **5**, 281–315.

Roter, D. (1979). Altering patient behaviour in interaction with providers. In *Research in Psychology and Medicine, Vol. 2*. (D. J. Oborne, M. M. Gruneberg and J. R. Eiser, eds). Academic Press, London.

Sackett, D. L., Haynes, R. B., Gibson, E. S., Hackett, B. C., Taylor, D. W., Roberts, R. S. and Johnson, A. L. (1975). Randomised clinical trial of strategies for improving medication compliance in primary hypertension. *Lancet* **1**, 1205–1207.

Skilbeck, C. E., Tulips, J. G. and Ley, P. (1977). The effects of fear arousal, fear position, fear exposure and sidedness on compliance with dietary instructions. *Eur. J. Soc. Psychol.* **7**, 221–239.

Spelman, M. A. and Ley, P. (1966). Knowledge of lung cancer and smoking habits. *Br. J. Soc. Clin. Psychol.* **5**, 207–210.

Spelman, M. S., Ley, P. and Jones, C. C. (1966). How do we improve doctor–patient communication in our hospitals. *World Hospitals* **2**, 126–134.

Suveges, L. (1977). The impact of counselling by the pharmacist on patient knowledge and compliance. *Proceedings of the McMaster Symposium on Compliance with Therapeutic Regimens*. McMaster University, Hamilton, Ontario.

Weibert, R. T. (1977). Potential distribution problems. *Drug Inform. J.* **11**, Special Supplement, 45s–48s.

5 Health Beliefs in the Consultation

Jennifer King

1 INTRODUCTION

"Disease may be a medical entity but illness is a social phenomenon" (Suchman, 1970). The idea that disease does not just occur in a vacuum but is dealt with in many different ways by different individuals is becoming increasingly evident both in medical research and practice. Detailed investigation of this has constituted a major contribution to the discussion of doctor–patient relationships. The introduction of sociology into medicine, together with terms such as "illness behaviour", "sick role" and "patient needs" has further strengthened the case for change in the doctor's role. In particular, rates of compliance with medical advice have become disturbingly low, with as much as half the advice not being taken up (Ley, 1974). The medical profession itself has produced critiques of the approach of doctors (Balint, 1976; Byrne and Long, 1976; Cohen, 1979). But although the problems of compliance are well-documented they are not completely understood.

Since the major causes of death today are ischaemic heart disease, stroke, cancer and accidents in the young, they are essential targets for prevention. But patients often fail to comply with advice about prevention. Each of these causes of death has at least some clearly identifiable risk factors. Smoking is the most prevalent followed by diet, stress and alcohol. These risk factors are often associated with a psychological dependence, or with firmly rooted health beliefs which fail to recognize or accept that any risk is involved. Health beliefs are often resistant to change, but not immutable. In order to persuade a patient to adopt more positive health behaviour, the doctor needs to obtain cooperation and compliance, often over a long period of time. This may involve a variety of actions by the patient, some of which may involve changes in lifestyle, and which involve taking personal responsibility for his or her own health.

Poor compliance with recommended advice has the effect of disrupting any potential benefits of preventive (or curative) advice. It also makes it impossible to estimate the effects of particular treatments or their potential value. Finally, it interferes with the doctor–patient relationship, by causing dissatisfaction with care leading back, in a vicious circle, to non-compliance. Psychological research over the last ten years has made significant advances towards explaining this low compliance. Previous research concentrated upon characteristics of the doctor which were found to affect the communication process between doctor and patient. Very little was known, however, about the factors in the patient which governed the decision to follow recommended advice. Recent research has emphasized the individual, subjective health beliefs of the patient, as well as several social and demographic characteristics thought to influence both attitudes and behaviour. The old medical model has become obsolete, being based on the erroneous assumption that there is a natural and automatic progression from information to attitudes to behaviour.

It would seem therefore, that disease management should be moving beyond a purely clinical approach, and should emphasize the psychosocial aspects of illness and patient health behaviour. This chapter will attempt to explore in some detail some of the reasons behind non-compliance. It will be shown how a psychological rather than a clinical approach can be applied to medical care. The chapter will attempt to suggest how doctor–patient communication and compliance might considerably be improved by greater consideration of social and psychological factors in the patient: in particular patient health beliefs. Finally, a counselling model will be proposed, based on patient health beliefs, and which may be applied to any consultations in which patients need to be persuaded to modify their behaviour.

It should be pointed out that this chapter has not attempted to include an exhaustive review of the research in this area, but instead has selected the most relevant and significant studies for this discussion.

2 THE PROBLEM OF NON COMPLIANCE

2.1 Patient Knowledge

The use of the term "health knowledge" is here being applied to knowledge of health-related issues, either directly concerned with illness or with "positive" health practices. Few studies exist which actually measure the extent of health knowledge, and those that have been reported provide limited information. Boyle (1970) studied very basic knowledge, and demonstrated a marked discrepancy between patient and doctor knowledge of the anatomical position of major organs and the definition of commonly used medical terms. Cole (1979) administered test words from printed health education materials to 120 patients and students to assess their medical vocabulary knowledge. It was apparent that many respondents had problems with the words, in particular patients of low social class. A detailed American survey on medical vocabulary knowledge (Samora *et al.*, 1961) found two-thirds of the respondents gave "inadequate" responses, and more than half failed to recognize four of the words: respiratory, cardiac, malignant and secretions. They also found that age and sex were not significantly associated with level of health knowledge; education appeared to be the most important factor.

Unfortunately, the relationship between patient knowledge and compliance is by no means clear. McKinley (1975) divided his subjects into "utilisers" and "under-utilisers" of medical care. It was found that the former had a consistently higher level of comprehension of medical words than the latter. The results obtained by Sackett *et al.* (1978) in a study of the role of increased knowledge in improving medication compliance amongst hypertensives, typify the usual findings in this area. Patient knowledge at intake was not associated with compliance; and although a group that was given intensive instruction subsequently demonstrated greater knowledge than the control group, compliance in both groups remained about the same. In summary, as Podell (1975) notes in his review: "At least a dozen studies show a positive association between patient knowledge and compliance. On the other hand, at least two dozen studies show no such relationship".

It seems reasonable to conclude that patient knowledge about certain essential details of medical advice is neither necessary nor sufficient for correct compliance. For individuals who are motivated to comply but lack sufficient knowledge of the correct procedures, information should be beneficial. If, however, a patient has some knowledge but is not sufficiently motivated additional information is unlikely to promote compliance. Clearly, then, it is necessary to investigate other factors which may influence patient compliance.

2.2 Doctor–Patient Communication

The literature on doctor–patient communication is very extensive and beyond the limits of this chapter. The chapter by Pendleton (see Chapter 1, this volume), reviews extensive evidence which shows that the consultation between doctor and patient needs to possess certain specific elements in order to achieve both satisfaction and subsequent compliance. Once again, however, it must be concluded that many of these elements constitute prerequisites which are essential for compliance and effective treatment, but still are not sufficient predictors of positive health behaviour. The tenuous link between knowledge and action is well-documented (Warren and Jahoda, 1973). It is evident, therefore, that doctors need to impart to most patients something more than just basic information. Perhaps we should benefit at this point, by moving towards a consideration of the characteristics of the patient, rather than those of the doctor and show how these are equally significant in the analysis of compliance.

2.3 Demographic Characteristics

Early research in behavioural science related compliance to easily identifiable dimensions, such as the demographic, social and personal characteristics of patients. These included age, sex, income, occupation, education and ethnic group. Studies used different measures of socio-economic status (SES), as well as very different medical conditions, patient populations and settings. The results of this research are therefore contradictory and inconclusive. With this in mind, it is worth pointing out a few findings in this area, simply because they often indicate the significance of other factors related to social class, which may have some bearing upon preventive health behaviour.

In a large American study, Coburn and Pope (1974) found that education, age, income and social participation (in that order) were the best predictors of preventive health behaviour. These factors were less important, however, when the recency of illness, and the distance from the patient's usual source of care were also taken into account.

Other studies have suggested that the relationship between SES and health behaviour is spurious (Steele and McBroom, 1972), and that the important factor is social integration—that is, the level of involvement with other people (Moody and Gray, 1973). It has been found that, in general, members of closely-knit, ethnocentric community, or similar family groups, tend to have less factual knowledge about medicine and (perhaps more significant) higher suspicion of professional medical care (Suchman, 1972). They tend, therefore, to rely on their own group for advice, and for help during illness. Although these particular findings came from an American study, a British study on community norms during pregnancy reached similar conclusions (Baric and MacArthur, 1979). Mothers' smoking, eating and drinking habits during pregnancy tended to conform to the expectations of their community, rather than to professional advice. This was not however, dependent on social class, suggesting that community influence is significant right across the social spectrum. Perhaps one of the most extensive studies of social class and health behaviour is the work by McKinlay (1972) on the use of health services in the

U.S.A. He found that those patients who made least use of health services appeared to sustain a "crisis existence" and tended, therefore, to be from the lower social classes. Despite the mass of conflicting findings in the whole area of social class and health, one significant fact still remains: "Lower class life is crisis life, constantly trying to make do with string where rope is needed" (Rainwater, 1968). This is highly significant not only to the way in which a doctor communicates with the patient, as we have already mentioned, but also to the type of strategy employed by a doctor to modify a patient's behaviour. A study by Pendleton *et al.* (1982) found that one in five consultations was reported to possess some element of communication difficulty. One of the significant factors causing such difficulties was the patient's social class. Such a finding may have several explanations—the following is often found to be significant. The term "prevention" involves a strong notion of the future, and indeed so do many kinds of treatment which last a long period of time. The problem faced by doctors has been vividly described by Muir Gray:

> The practitioners of preventive medicine mostly experience a social and temporal reality which stretches decades into the future, while those at whom their messages are principally directed, because they have higher mobility and mortality rates, experience a reality in which the future finishes next Friday. (Gray, 1979, p. 144)

In addition to the consideration of time, there is also the question of the impersonal nature of much medical treatment and health education. For example, many patients are often given statistics about smokers dying from lung cancer, or pregnant mothers are told how many other mothers have had premature births through smoking during pregnancy. Despite the evidence on the influence of community norms, facts and figures about other people can be irrelevant and often inappropriate. For example, the classic argument of a smoking pregnant mother is often: "I smoked through my last pregnancy and my baby was alright". She may, of course, use the same argument about a friend or family member, but statistics about anyone outside her immediate social world will often be seen as irrelevant. Instead, a patient needs to be told about the personal risk and consequences associated with illness or particular habit such as smoking, as well as being given treatment which will be appropriate for that particular patient: one that will involve few personal costs and emphasize benefits which are appealing to the individual concerned. The questions of subjective estimates of risk, costs and benefits will be covered in greater detail below.

It is evident from the research that no simple relationship exists between demographic factors and either compliance or any other kind of preventive behaviour. The only general consistency seems to be the association between non-compliance and medication errors, and extremes of age. Social class factors may be compared to risk factors, in the sense that they help to identify groups or individuals who tend not to comply, but they do not reveal exactly how this compliance might best be achieved. We cannot account, moreover, for the substantial numbers of patients who possess one or more of these adverse characteristics, but who comply nonetheless. An analysis of compliance based only on social class does not provide a unified conceptual explanation. It can only be concluded that non-compliance is commonly found among patients of all demographic, personality and social types.

It is, nevertheless, apparent from other lines of research that social class does play an important part in patient cooperation and compliance. Research has tended to concentrate on the type of social class *per se*, usually identified by education and income, rather than the implications of working class life for health behaviour. It is suggested that these are highly significant in the doctor–patient relationship, and ultimately to the success or failure of treatment. But many other psychological concepts, some of which have already been hinted at, would appear to be far more valuable in predicting a patient's health behaviour. Until this point, the emphasis has been mainly upon factors in the doctor, and objective characteristics of the patient. We need to move to a consideration of the subjective perceptions of the patient, and ultimately to show that these may be just as crucial to the doctor–patient relationship as any of the other factors discussed.

3 PATIENT HEALTH BELIEFS

3.1 The Health Belief Model

We can assume that a patient's decision to accept or reject medical advice is motivated by more than just objective knowledge, or even the personal characteristics of the doctor. There can be little doubt as to the importance of these factors, but they still do not supply the whole story. It has become evident from a wealth of research over the last decade that different patients see health and illness in many different ways. A patient will not always accept an objective medical explanation or diagnosis at face value. This acceptance may be coloured by many personal beliefs held by the patient. It is motivation which translates the health belief into behaviour, and which therefore needs to be identified by the doctor.

The most extensively validated model of patient's health behaviour is the Health Belief Model (Becker; 1974; Rosenstock, 1974; Maiman and Becker, 1974; Becker and Maiman, 1975; Becker *et al.*, 1977) (Fig. 5.1) which actually identifies some of these motivational factors. Based on a well-established body of psychological theory, the model was originally developed to explain and predict preventive health actions such as immunization, attendance at screenings, and dental care. It has also, however, been used to explain compliance relative to seeking diagnosis and following prescribed medication, dietary and other types of advice. The model contains the following main elements:

(i) Health Motivation: an individual's degree of interest in, and concern about health matters.

(ii) Susceptibility: perceived vulnerability (or resusceptibility) to the particular illness, including acceptance of the diagnosis.

(iii) Severity: perceptions concerning the probable seriousness of the consequences of contracting the illness or leaving it untreated. Consequences may be organic and/or social.

(iv) Benefits and costs: the individual's estimate of the benefits of taking recommended health action, weighed against the costs or barriers involved. Such costs might include for example financial expense, physical and/or emotional discomfort, or possible side effects.

(v) Cue to actions: something must occur to "trigger" these perceptions and lead to the appropriate health behaviour. This stimulus can be either internal (such as symptoms), or external (such as magazine articles, a reminder from the doctor, or illness in the family).

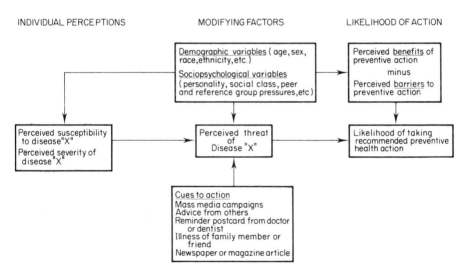

Fig. 5.1.   The original health belief model (after Becker and Maiman, 1975).

The significant point about the elements in the Health Belief Model is that they are the person's subjective perceptions of the situation rather than objective medical facts. As such, they are open to many sources of bias and misconception. The advantage, however, is that the individual's perceptions are often amenable to modification. The Health Belief Model also derives much of its strength from the fact that it does not rely on characteristics like social class or vague allusions to global attitudes, to explain or predict compliance. It rests on the predictive value of the individual's health beliefs and perceptions.

In order to illustrate exactly how comprehensive and useful this model can be, some of its main elements will be discussed in more detail, with a view to demonstrating how these concepts might usefully be incorporated into the general practice consultation.

3.1.1 *Perceived Susceptibility*

A considerable number of studies have demonstrated a positive relationship between a person's subjective estimate of personal vulnerability and compliance with medical advice. Some examples of these are screening for cervical (Kegeles, 1969), breast (Fink *et al.*, 1972) or other cancer (Haefner and Kirscht, 1970), for tuberculosis (Hochbaum, 1958), heart disease (Haefner and Kirscht, 1970), and for dental problems (Kegeles, 1963) and immunizations (Katatsky, 1977) against various illnesses. The concept of perceived vulnerability has also been applied to contraceptive compliance (Rosenstock *et al.*, 1959). Although it has been argued that pregnancy cannot be regarded as a disease and that therefore the Health Belief Model is inappropriate in this case, others have argued that the model need not be limited to preventive actions against undesirable conditions, and that ultimately it is the motivation of the person which is an important determinant in any form of preventive action (Fisher, 1977).

In examining the relationship between perceived vulnerability and taking prescribed medication, the concept of resusceptibility has been used, as some diagnosis of illness has already been made. For example, significant positive associations have been found between a mother's belief in the possibility of her child contracting rheumatic fever again, and compliance both in administering the penicillin and clinic attendance (Elling *et al.*, 1960). Similar findings are illustrated in studies of mothers of children with otitis media, and mothers of obese children (Becker *et al.*, 1977). Mothers compliance with recommended treatment depended upon their feeling that the child was resusceptible to the present illness, their belief in the accuracy of the diagnosis, and their perception that the child was easily susceptible to disease (Fig. 5.2).

3.1.2 *Perceptions of severity*

The findings on the relation between perceived seriousness and preventive

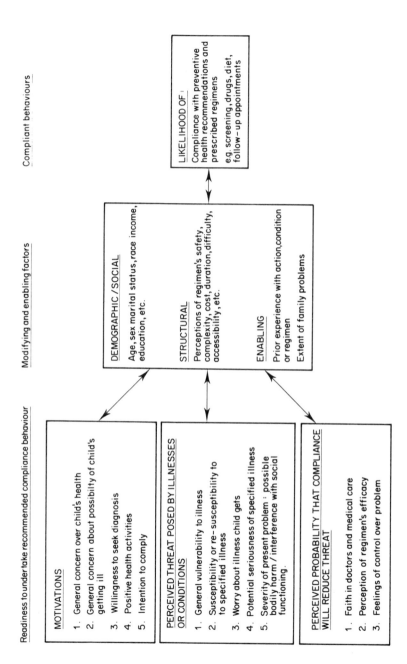

Fig. 5.2. Model for predicting and explaining mother's compliance behaviours (after "The health belief model", Becker, *et al.*, 1927).

health behaviour are not quite so conclusive. This factor has been found significantly to influence compliance only with certain health recommendations: for example dental care (Tash *et al.*, 1969), preventing an accident (Suchman, 1967), seeking care in response to symptoms (Battistella, 1971), initiating actions to prevent coronary heart disease (Campbell, 1971), and bringing a child to the clinic for preventive care (Becker *et al.*, 1977).

No significant associations were found, however, between perceptions of seriousness and participation in several types of screening programmes, or for accepting immunizations. Recent interpretation of these findings suggests that, for the asymptomatic person, very low levels of severity are not sufficiently motivating whereas very high levels actually inhibit action (Leventhal, 1965). Thus, both extremes are associated with low likelihood of taking preventive health action. Leventhal *et al.* (1965), have concluded that once a person has reached some subjective level of fear, it is unlikely that any increase in perceived severity will encourage compliance. Too little fear inhibits action, but so does too much fear. The same is true of anxiety (Gray, 1979). If a smoker, for example, cannot reduce the risk of illness and therefore the anxiety by stopping smoking, then he or she may choose to reduce the anxiety by use of a defence mechanism. Another example in which a high level of perceived seriousness may inhibit action delay is seeking screening for cancer. Studies demonstrate that it is often fear of the result, and the consequent distress on discovering cancer, which cause people to avoid screening. In a study on women's ability to perform breast self-examination, it was found that only when women were convinced of the benefits of early detection of breast cancer were they likely to carry out this test (Manfredi *et al.*, 1977). If however, too great an emphasis was placed on the dangers of breast cancer, in the absence of convincing information about the benefits of regular screening, this promoted fear and tension, thus inhibiting the ability to learn these self-examination techniques.

These findings have important implications for doctor–patient relations. It seems clear that a certain level of fear and anxiety must be induced in order to promote some preventive action (Ley, 1978). This was clearly demonstrated in a study in which people with prior family experience with symptoms tended to express less inclination to seek prompt medical care (Banks and Keller, 1971). One possible explanation for this is that knowledge gained from prior personal experience of symptoms reduces uncertainty and therefore also reduces anxiety, and this diminishes motivation from immediate medical attention. But at the same time it is important for the doctor to offer some means of reducing it immediately, if this is at all possible, since delay often increases tension. It is, in other words, not only the type of threat and perceived seriousness which affects the patient, but the kind of action proposed to relieve the tension. One of the problems with over-zealous health educators is their excessive emphasis upon danger without accompanying this with constructive action.

3.1.3 *Perceptions of Benefits and Costs*

In many instances of preventive health behaviour, compliance cannot be predicted solely on the basis of either perceived vulnerability or severity. There are cases in which an individual may see himself or herself as highly vulnerable to an illness and recognize that the consequences will be serious, but still may not follow the recommended course of action, simply because the costs of taking this particular action are too high. Often, this does not mean simply financial costs, although in the case of, for example, hypertension treatment this may be a significant barrier. More often, however, the costs may be psychological, as we have already discussed. The costs of a particular treatment may also be high in terms of side effects or discomfort. Indeed, perceived costs have been measured in a variety of ways, although several factors have been dependable predictors of noncompliance. For example, regardless of the person's concern over the dangers of polio he or she will not obtain the recommended vaccine if the safety of the vaccine is at all in doubt (Katatsky, 1977). Haynes concludes that:

> A steep gradient has been demonstrated in which the compliance exhibited by patients who must acquire new habits, such as taking medications, is much greater than that exhibited by those who must alter old behaviours such as dietary or vocational habits, which in turn exceeds that of those who must break personal habits such as smoking or drinking or nonmedical use of drugs. (Haynes, 1976)

There are also significant findings in terms of the effects of the doctor–patient communication on compliance, discussed by Ley, but which can also constitute an important example of a perceived cost involved in preventive behaviour (Coe and Wessen, 1965). Also found to influence patient cooperation are barriers in the form of client dissatisfaction with certain aspects of the way in which the organization provides medical care. For example, compliance appears to be better where continuity of care is provided (Gordis *et al.*, 1971). This is perhaps due to the enhancing effect of a regular doctor– patient contact on health beliefs; partly because of the effect of the doctor "checking-up" on the patient's behaviour.

One of the most commonly perceived benefits of preventive health action is the effectiveness of the treatment. As was demonstrated in the study on breast (BSE) self-examination, the likelihood that mothers would perform BSE was enhanced by the women's beliefs in the efficacy of self-examination, and by the belief that early detection would lead to a more favourable prognosis. Perceived benefits need not, however, be simply in terms of the efficacy of medication, but also of professional medical care and intervention. Once again, therefore, effective communication between doctor and patient is often a highly valued benefit of medical treatment.

3.1.4 *Cues to Action*

Something must arouse a patient's perception of threat before that perception can actually lead to preventive behaviour; this stimulus can be either internal, such as symptoms, or external, such as a magazine article, illness in the family, contact with health professionals (Rosenstock, 1975), or simply a reminder card from the doctor. Although these particular cues are not, in themselves, psychological processes, they are often important "triggers" to such processes. Alternatively, they might also be responsible for translating a belief into action. If, for example, a patient already recognizes the potential threat of an illness, a reminder card from the doctor might be all that is needed to encourage the patient actually to do something about his or her condition.

3.2 Limitations of the Health Belief Model.

Firstly, for the Health Belief Model to be useful, all its factors need to be considered—and it is often only the interaction between these that can predict health behaviour.

Secondly, there has been no research on the stability of the model's major variables over time. For example, perceived risk may be more salient during one period of time.

Thirdly, there has been no research into the conditions under which the health beliefs were acquired. This is a more crucial consideration for doctor–patient communication. What are the determinants of these patient health beliefs? Why does one patient see himself as more vulnerable than another, to a particular illness? How does the patient come to see himself or herself as susceptible in the first place? How does a person come to believe a specific action is preventive? What governs the desire for a particular level of health? In other words we know very little of the psychological processes which govern these beliefs. Chapter 7 in this volume by Jaspars *et al.* discusses these ideas in more detail. Nevertheless, despite these criticisms, the Health Belief model remains the best model of preventive health behaviour proposed to date.

4 USING HEALTH BELIEFS IN THE CONSULTATION

It is apparent from the research that patient beliefs are often highly idiosyncratic, making it extremely difficult to devise one educational prescription suitable for all patients. Discovering these beliefs are, however, essential for persuading a patient to adopt more positive health behaviour. Indeed, considerable persuasion is often necessary for a patient to alter a lifelong pattern of behaviour. Many doctors are unable to structure their consultations in such a way as to have a significant impact on health behaviour. They also would argue, moreover, that time constraints of the consultation make it impractical to attempt to elicit individual beliefs about a particular action or treatment. With these considerations in mind a counselling model has been devised, which is described below.

It is important to note firstly, that this model is designed specifically for consultations in which the doctor wants to persuade a patient to modify his or her behaviour. As such, it is particularly appropriate in health education consultations, as opposed to curative clinical medicine. Secondly, it should be pointed out that most consultations probably contain part of the proposed technique, although the whole model is rarely used, either consciously or systematically. Finally, the model does not attempt to be exhaustive or foolproof: it simply attempts to present a structured framework or "check-list" on which to base health education, and which can plausibly be fitted into the average consultation time. Ideally, the elements of the model should be used in the order presented below, although naturally this is flexible. The model will be illustrated by the example of a doctor trying to persuade a pregnant mother to stop smoking (King and Eiser, 1982; Pendleton and King, 1980).

(1) *Elicit the patient's health beliefs.* This means finding out the mother's beliefs about smoking in general, and more specifically, the effects of smoking on her unborn baby.

(2) *Reinforce* any statements made by the patient which may indicate motivation towards health. In this case, reinforce statements consistent with a reduction of smoking for the sake of the baby.

(3) *Counter* any expressed "myths" on the subject held to be true by the patient.

(4) *Inform* the patient about the actual risks and severity of her behaviour. Also inform her about the costs involved in altering her behaviour, but strongly counterbalanced by the benefits—in this case, a healthier baby.

(5) *Plan* with the patient, a preventive course of action which will be appropriate to her individual needs and lifestyle.

(6) *Terminate* the consultation with a specific objective (e.g. to reduce the number of cigarettes smoked to five a day by the next visit).

(7) *Follow-up* with regular interviews to reinforce advice and to provide continuous support.

Clearly, this type of approach goes far beyond the "scaremongering" tactics of describing to the mother the dangers of smoking during pregnancy; and also takes into account individual needs and attitudes, allowing both flexibility and structure within the consultation, and also in the resulting advice. Above all it is a supportive and constructive strategy, rather than being dogmatic or punitive. Many doctors will already do some of these things very well, but it may require some additional skill to use the whole model effectively. As several chapters in this volume suggest, such skills can be learned to considerable effect, with appropriate training.

5 SUMMARY AND CONCLUSIONS

It is evident from this discussion that, in order to increase patient compliance and the effectiveness of medical intervention, the doctor needs to do far more than impart basic information concerning the prescribed treatment. This research on health beliefs shows that patients' attitudes towards risk, severity and so on, are important predictors of behaviour, but only under certain conditions or at certain levels. Frequently, health behaviour results from a combination of different beliefs. The various studies show that, of people who do not follow recommended advice, some are unmotivated, some lack beliefs in their vulnerability to an illness, while others fail to see the benefits of a proposed course of action. These individual differences make the doctor's task in increasing compliance even more daunting, as it suggests that there is no single persuasive strategy suitable for all patients. Research findings to date leave little doubt, however, as to the crucial importance of eliciting the patient's health beliefs. This has the added advantage of promoting a more personal communication between doctor and patient, thus strengthening their relationship and possibly increasing compliance because of the greater satisfaction of the patient. Having elicited these health beliefs, they need to be translated into action. A counselling model has been proposed for the express purpose of persuading patients to modify their behaviour. The strategy is essentially supportive, and provides the kind of structured approach to health education which has so far been lacking in general practice.

In summary, preventive health behaviour has been too often discussed in a "medical-scientific" context. Not enough attention has been focused on individuals as producers of health as a commodity, rather than consumers of health care services. It is strongly recommended, therefore, that doctors move beyond a purely clinical approach to the psychosocial factors that influence health behaviour. It is particularly important that this type of approach be incorporated into the curricula of medical training. This may increase the number of doctors committed to prevention as well as to treatment, and ultimately lead to patients accepting greater responsibility for their own health.

REFERENCES

Balint, M. (1957). *The Doctor, His Patient and the Illness*. Tavistock, London.

Banks, F. R. and Keller, M. D. (1971). Symptom experience and health action. *Med. Care* **9**, 498–503.

Baric, L. and MacArthur, C. (1979). Exploration of health norms in pregnancy. *Br. J. Soc. Prev. Med.*

Battistella, R. M. (1971). Factors associated with delay in the initiation of physicians' care among late adulthood persons. *Am. J. Pub. Hlth* **61**, 1348–1361.

Becker, M. H. (1974). The Health Belief Model and Personal Health Behaviour. *Health Ed. Monog.* **2**, 328–335.

Becker, M. H. and Maiman, L. A. (1975). Sociobehavioural determinants of compliance with medical care recommendations. *Med. Care.* **13**, 10–24.

Becker, M. H., Maiman, L. A., Kirscht, J. P., Haefner, D. P. and Drachman, R. H. (1977a). The Health Belief Model and prediction of dietary compliance. A field experiment. *J. Hlth Soc. Behav.* **18**, 348–366.

Becker, M. H., Nathanson, C. A., Drachman, R. H. and Kirscht, J. P. (1977b). Mothers' health beliefs and children's clinic visits. A prospective study. *J. Comm. Hlth* **3**, 125–135.

Becker, M., Haefner, D., Kasl, S., Kirscht, J., Maiman, L. and Rosenstock, I. (1977c). Selected psychosocial models and correlates of individual health-related behaviours. *Med. Care* **15**, 27–46.

Boyle, C. (1970). Differences between patients' and doctors' interpretations of some common medical terms. *Br. Med. J.* **2**, 286–9.

Byrne, P. and Long, B. (1976). *Doctors Talking to Patients*. H.M.S.O., London.

Campbell, D. A. (1971). A study of the preventive health behaviour of a group of men with increased risk for the development of coronary heart disease. Ph.D. dissertation, Ohio State University.

Coburn, D. and Pope, C. (1974). Socioeconomic status and preventive health behaviour. *J. Hlth Soc. Behav.* **15**, 67.

Coe, R. M. and Wessen, A. (1965). Social psychological factors in influencing the use of community health resources. *Am. J. Pub. Hlth* **55**, 1024.

Cohen, S. J. (1979). *New Directions in Patient Compliance*. Lexington Books, New York.

Cole, R. (1979). The understanding of medical terminology used in printed health education materials. *Health Ed. J.* **38**, 111–121.

Elling, R., Whittemore, R. and Green, M. (1960). Patient participation in a pediatric program. *J. Hlth Hum. Behav.* **1**, 183–191.

Fink, R., Shapiro, S. and Roester, R. (1972). Impact of efforts to increase participation in repetitive screenings for early breast cancer detection. *Am. J. Publ. Hlth* **62**, 328–336.

Fisher, A. A. (1977). The Health Belief Model and contraceptive behaviour: limits to the application of a conceptual framework. *Health Ed. Monog.* **5**, 244–250.

Gordis, L., Markowitz, M. and Lilienfield, A. M. (1971). Evaluation of the effectiveness of comprehensive care in influencing infant health. *Pediatrics* **48**, 766.

Gray, M. (1979). *Man Against Disease: Preventive Medicine.* Oxford University Press, Oxford.

Haefner, D. and Kirscht, J. P. (1970). Motivational and behavioural effects of modifying health beliefs. *Pub. Hlth Reps* **85**, 478–484.

Haynes, R. B. (1976). A critical review of the "determinants" of patient compliance with therapeutic regimens. In *Compliance with Therapeutic Regimens*, (D. L. Sackett and R. B. Haynes, eds), pp. 26–39. John Hopkins University Press, Baltimore.

Hochbaum, G. M. (1958). Public Participation in Medical Screening programs. A socio-psychological study. Pub. Health. Service Publication 572. Washington D.C. Government Printing Office, 1958.

Katatsky, M. E. (1977). The Health Belief Model as a conceptual framework for explaining contraceptive compliance. *Health Ed. Monog.* **5**, 232–243.

Kegeles, S. S. (1963). Some motives for seeking preventive dental care. *J. Am. Dental Assoc.* **67**, 90–98.

Kegeles, S. S. (1969). A field experiment attempt to change beliefs and behaviour of women in an urban ghetto. *J. Hlth Soc. Behav.* **10**, 115–124.

King, J. B. and Eiser, J. R. (1981). A strategy for counselling pregnant smokers. *Health Ed. J.* **40**(3).

Leventhal, H. (1965). Fear communications in the acceptance of preventive health practices. *Bull New York Acad. Med.* **41**, 144–1168.

Leventhal, H., Singer, R. and Jones, S. (1965). The effects of fear and specificity of recommendations. *J. Pers. Soc. Psych.* **2**, 20–25.

Ley, P. (1974). Communication in the clinical setting. *Br. J. Orthodont.* **1**, 173.

Ley, P. (1978). Psychological and behavioural factors in weight loss. In *Recent Advances in Obesity Research, 2* (G. A. Bray, ed.). Newman Publishing, London.

McKinlay, J. B. (1972). Some approaches and problems in the study of the use of services—an overview. *J. Hlth Soc. Behav.* **13**, 115.

McKinley, J. (1975). Who is really ignorant—physician or patient? *J. Hlth Soc. Behav.* **16**, (1), 3.

Maiman, L. A. and Becker, M. H. (1974). The Health Belief Model: Origins and correlates in psychological theory. *Health Ed. Monog.* **2**, 336–353.

Manfredi, C., Warnecke, R. B., Graham, S. and Rosenthal, S. (1977). Social psychological correlates of health behaviour. Knowledge of breast self examination techniques among black women. *Soc. Sci. Med.* **11**, 433–440.

Moody, P. and Gray, R. (1973). Social class, social integration and the use of preventive health services. In *Patients, Physicians and Illness* (Jaco, ed.) 3rd Ed.

Pendleton, D. A. and King, J. B. (1980). Doctor–patient communication. The medium and the message. *Oxford Med. Sch. Gazette* **31**, 30–32.

Pendleton, D. A., Jaspars, J. M. F. and Tate, P. (1982). Doctor–Patient Communication: Difficulties Reported by Doctors (in press).

Podell, R. N. (1975). *Physician's Guide to Compliance in Hypertension West Point.* Merck, Pennsylvania.

Rainwater, L. (1968). The lower class: Health, illness and medical institutions. In *Among the People* (Deutscher and Thompson, eds). p. 260.

Rosenstock, I. L. (1974). Historical Origins of the Health Belief Model: Origins and correlates in psychological theory. *Health Ed. monog.* **2**, 336–353.

Rosenstock, I. M. (1975). Patients compliance with health regimens. *J. Am. Med. Assoc.* **234**, 402–403.

Rosenstock, I. M., Derryberry, M. and Carriger, B. K. (1959). Why people fail to seek poliomyelitis vaccination. *Pub. Hlth Reps* **74**, 98–103.

Sackett, D. L., Haynes, R. B., Gibson, E. S., Taylor, D. W., Roberts, R. S. and Johnson, A. L. (1978). Patient Compliance with Antihypertensive Regimens. Patient Counselling and Health Education, 1, 18–21.

Samora, J., Saunders, L. and Larson, R. (1961). Medical vocabulary knowledge among hospital patients. *J. Hlth Hum. Behav.* **2**, 83.

Steele, J. L. and McBroom, W. H. (1972). Conceptual and empirical dimensions of health behaviour. *J. Hlth Soc. Behav.* **13**, 382.

Suchman, E. A. (1967). Preventive health behaviour. A model for research on community health campaigns. *J. Hlth Soc. Behav.* **8**, 197–209.

Suchman, E. A. (1970). Health attitudes and Behaviour. *Arch. Env.tal Health* **20**, 105

Suchman, E. (1972). Social patterns of illness and medical care. In *Patients, Physicians and Illness* (Jaco, ed.) 2nd Ed.

Tash, R. H., O'Shea, R. M. and Cohen, L. K. (1969). Testing a preventive symptomatic theory of dental health behaviour. *Am. J. Pub. Hlth* **59**, 514–521.

Warren, N. and Jahoda, M. (eds) (1973) *Attitudes*. Penguin Books, Harmondsworth.

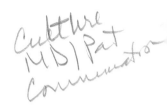

6 Doctors, Patients and their Cultures

Stephen Bochner

A medical consultation is a special instance of a social encounter, at least until the day when patients take their aches and pains to a computer rather than a human doctor. The advantage of considering the medical consultation from the point of view of its social psychology, is that it can be placed within a general body of knowledge about human interaction. In particular, the principles that underly interpersonal episodes (Harré, 1977) can be used to provide an account of the transactions that occur between doctors and patients.

Research in social psychology (e.g. Secord and Backman, 1964) has established that when two or more persons interact with each other, their behaviour is greatly influenced by how they define their own and one another's roles. These definitions include the mutual expectations that they bring to the encounter, that is, what they believe is expected of them and what they can legitimately expect of the other person, *in that particular context*. What is being stressed here is that the mutual rights and obligations of participants in a particular encounter are very much situation bound (Argyle *et al.*, 1981). In the general practice consultation, patients expect certain actions from their doctors, and doctors expect certain actions from their patients, the behaviour of each party being related to the special purpose of their coming together. In another context, say when a doctor and a patient meet at a social function held at the home of a mutual acquaintance, a different set of rules apply.

1 MISUNDERSTANDINGS IN EVERYDAY LIFE

Work on communication difficulties by social psychologists has suggested several general principles that underly the misunderstandings that only too often create havoc among people engaged in some joint enterprise. It should be emphasized that the present analysis is not about "difficult" people, or scoundrels deceiving each other. The discussion, as the sub-heading implies, centres on the pitfalls that face reasonable people of good will, trying to exchange views with other reasonable people of equally good will. Some of the main principles of miscommunication will now be listed, and related to the doctor–patient meeting.

2 ROLE UNCERTAINTY

Role uncertainty exists when the parties are unclear about their own and the other person's legitimate expectations and obligations. For example, when doctors ask their patients if they are in pain, the doctor may expect the patient to report any and all pain felt. However, the patient may think the question relates to the presenting symptom only, mentioning the painful throat but remaining silent about the throbbing knee joint. On a more complex level, the patient may not perceive that the doctor has a dual responsibility, one to the patient and the other to society. The latter may lead to a reluctance in prescribing certain drugs which in the physician's opinion ought to be reserved for serious cases. Perhaps the doctor may think twice about ordering expensive treatment that is publicly funded, or refuse to issue certificates in borderline cases, all actions which the patient may misunderstand and resent. On the other side, physicians may not fully realize when patients expect more than just medication from their doctors, that often what patients really want is reassurance, advice or just someone to talk to.

3 ROLE NON-CORRESPONDENCE

Role non-correspondence occurs when both parties are quite quite clear about what they want and expect from a relationship, but fail to agree about their mutual rights and obligations. For example, some patients may not see why they should disclose to their doctors who their sexual contacts are, a perennial problem in the epidemiology of venereal disease. Doctors, for their part may not wish to become involved in marital disputes, or in making life and death decisions, or in industrial issues between management and trade unions. More commonly, patients may demand information that their doctors will refuse to give on the grounds that such knowledge in the possession of the patient may be dangerous or harmful. Many busy doctors also take the view that it is not their job to provide reassurance, advice, or a sympathetic ear, and explicitly reject the overtures of patients who are excessively dependent, anxious or lonely. In effect, role non-correspondence places the parties into an attitude of unresolved conflict vis-à-vis each other. In many circumstances, even quite mild role conflict can reduce the satisfaction that each person would otherwise have derived from the encounter.

4 DEFINITION DISPARITY

Another source of interpersonal friction is when the participants define the situation differently, or attach different labels to salient aspects of the encounter. In the medical context, a good example is the frequently occurring disparity in the very definition of what constitutes illness and cure. Some patients, perhaps the majority, have a mechanical or chemical model of illness. These people liken their bodies to a machine that, like all mechanical devices, sometimes breaks down. When this unfortunate event occurs, the correct response is to treat the physical symptom with a physical remedy such as a pill or an operation. The prognosis will depend largely on the physical condition of the patient, and on the appropriateness and efficacy of the physical and chemical intervention. Some doctors, on the other hand, perhaps in the minority but nevertheless quite substantially represented in the profession, may entertain a psychosomatic or sociological model of illness, and follow the recommendation of the Royal College of General Practitioners (1972) that diagnoses should always be based on physical, psychological and social considerations. For these physicians, the correct procedure is to regard both the aetiology and the intervention in the context of the patient's life style and social relations, and may often imply no physical or chemical treatment whatsoever. There is no need to elaborate on the potential for confusion when a pill-swallowing patient encounters a sociologically inclined physician; or conversely, when a pill-pushing doctor is treating a patient who is convinced that all diseases are in the mind. Although the body–mind relationship is generally regarded as being in the province of the philosopher, it does have practical consequences for medicine, more so in psychiatry, which is outside the scope of this chapter, but also in the consulting rooms of the general practitioner.

5 GOAL DISPARITY

It is not uncommon to find that the aims of the participants in a social encounter differ substantially. This is clearly evident in instances where the parties have met explicitly for the purpose of negotiating, for example in labour-management conferences, or in legal procedures based on the adversary system. However, there are many situations where the goals of the participants differ markedly, but in a way that is unstated, unacknowledged, or even unrecognized by the persons concerned. Encounters between members of different ethnic groups are sometimes at cross purposes due to the hidden differences in the respective purposes of the participants. For example, some male students from certain parts of Southeast Asia, attending university in Australia, misunderstood the informality of Australian girls to be indicative of their availability for casual sexual intercourse, whereas the girls were simply expressing warmth and friendship to the visitors (Bochner and Wicks, 1972). As can be expected, many of these encounters were less than successful, with each person blaming the other for spoiling the relationship.

In the health care field, there may exist a disparity between the goal of providing immediate symptom relief, and the sometimes but not necessarily incompatible aim of effecting a permanent cure. This conflict is particularly evident in the field of dentistry, which tends to be divided between practitioners emphasizing preventive care, and those doing primarily restorative work (Bochner, in preparation). The same issue is not uncommonly encountered in the consulting rooms of the general practitioner, when the doctor may wish to improve the long-term health of the patient, only to realize that the sole concern of the sufferer is immediate relief from the presenting symptoms (Pendleton, 1981).

6 COMMUNICATION DIFFICULTIES AND CULTURE DISTANCE

Role uncertainty, role non-correspondence, definition disparity, and goal disparity may all operate below the level of the full awareness of one or both participants. In other words, in a medical consultation, neither the doctor nor the patient may be fully aware that they are operating at cross-purposes, although both parties are likely to feel uneasy about an interaction that is out of tune in terms of the concepts just reviewed. This suggests that it may be useful to regard the doctor–patient relationship from the same theoretical perspective as the analysis of inter-ethnic and inter-cultural communication difficulties. The most general statement of the problem is that communication effectiveness decreases as the distance between the respective cultures of the participants increases (Triandis, 1975). The advantage of this formulation is that the principle has great generality, and can therefore bring together a large set of apparently unrelated phenomena under the same theoretical umbrella. Not only is the idea true at the level of major cultural divisions, but it can also account for communication problems between sub-cultural groups. For example, viewed from this perspective, the so-called generation gap is really a division between two distinct sub-cultures, the adolescent peer group on the one hand, and the parental group on the other. These two groups may share more or less the same linguistic forms (or at least speak mutually intelligible dialects) but may have quite different expectations about what is appropriate behaviour. Some of the items of disagreement may include what are the correct clothes to wear in public, who can or cannot sleep with whom, what to spend one's money on, and the value or otherwise of hard work. And since culture is basically a shared set of assumptions, particularly in the realm of interpersonal conduct, the cultural gap between father and son is in principle no different from say the disparity between a Scottish and a New Guinea highlander. However, in the case of two people sharing the same language but belonging to different sub-groups, this only becomes clear when their communicating is viewed from the perspective of culture distance. Only then is it obvious that the principles governing relations between sub-cultures are the same as those affecting communication between major cultural groupings. It then becomes possible to apply the analysis and remedial practices used in the field of cross-cultural relations, to problems of communication between sub-groups within a particular society. The major divisions in most societies, and those known to affect communication across their boundaries, are age, social class, occupational specialization, educational level, and to a lesser extent sex, religion and political orientation.

In the past, the traditional response of English travellers trying to make themselves understood while abroad, was to speak a little louder, hardly the stuff of effective communication. However, since the end of World War II, with the demise of the colonial era and the emergence of a pluralistic, and yet at the same time closely inter-connected, global social system, a great deal of research has been conducted into the principles and practices of cross-cultural communication (for a review see Bochner, 1982). In the context of the present discussion, two conclusions in particular can be drawn from this work. The first has already been alluded to, and is the finding that quite often the participants in a cross-cultural encounter are unaware that they are sending unintended messages, and that they are distorting incoming information. The second point concerns remedial action, and is based on the central idea that to communicate effectively with other persons, it is not enough to know their language; we must also have a degree of familiarity with their culture. The two points are interrelated, and will now be discussed with reference to acquiring the social skills of a second culture.

7 CULTURE LEARNING

People learning a second culture include all those individuals who for one reason or another work, live, study, or play in a society other than the one they were brought up in (Bochner, 1982). The core curriculum of culture learning consists of the social skills employed in successfully negotiating the everyday encounters with members of the host society, in the work place, streets, shops, cafes and homes of the receiving country (Furnham and Bochner, 1982). The major obstacle, however, to learning another culture is that it is not usually readily accessible to a newcomer. A culture learner is by definition an outsider, and hence denied the sort of intimate contact with members of the host culture that insiders have. Moreover, some of the vital aspects of a culture, particularly in the realm of interpersonal relations, are hidden, highly subtle, and often not consciously articulated even by the insiders. This is particularly evident in the area of non-verbal communication (Argyle, 1982; Collett, 1982). Gestures, posture, eye gaze, tone of voice all communicate and are interpreted to have quite specific meanings, and yet quite often their impact may be below the threshold of awareness of the participants sending and receiving these signals. Thus if outsiders inquired about these aspects of the communication process, the participants might have difficulty in understanding the question or supplying the correct answer, even if they were inclined to do so.

Variations in time perspective provide another good example of the implicit nature of much communication, its cultural specificity, and the consequences of these variables on cross-cultural understanding. For instance, Levine *et al.* (1980) found that Americans tend to see a person who is never late for an appointment as more successful than someone who is occasionally late, who in turn is perceived as more successful than someone who is always late. Exactly the opposite is the case in Brazil, where arriving late for an appointment is indicative of success. The implication is that Americans may look down on Brazilians who arrive late for meetings, whereas Brazilians will have a poor opinion of Americans who arrive punctually. This does not augur well for any meetings attended by Americans and Brazilians unaware of the social conventions of each other's cultures. Only through the mutual knowledge of the conception of time and punctuality in America and Brazil could such misunderstanding be avoided, yet it is unlikely that such information will be acquired during the normal course of interaction. In effect, culture learning does not come naturally, but has to be systematically acquired, with the help of specially developed techniques and procedures (Brislin and Pedersen, 1976).

8 DOCTORS, PATIENTS, AND THEIR RESPECTIVE CULTURES

The excursion into the psychology of cross-cultural communication problems was made so as to provide a context for a new look at the doctor–patient relationship. The subsequent discussion is restricted to British doctors and British patients, since the empirical study illustrating the theoretical analysis was conducted in England. Any extensions to other medical settings will have to await further empirical elaboration.

The cross-cultural model of communication difficulties suggests the following hypotheses about how general practitioners and patients relate to each other. First, it is quite likely that in many instances, there will exist a cultural gap between the doctor and the patient. This hypothesis is derived from the demographic characteristics of the medical profession. Most doctors are middle-class males (although the proportion of female medical graduates is steadily increasing), and by definition all are highly educated in a very specialized discipline with its own concepts, language, ethics and world view. Each of these characteristics (class, sex, ideology, etc.) can be thought of as a set of assumptions that different patients share to varying degrees with their particular doctor. Thus each patient in theory can be located on a point on each of several continua, together constituting the cultural distance separating the doctor from the patient. Some of the continua may be more important than others, for example social class similarity-dissimilarity may have a bigger impact on communication effectiveness than say sex similarity; and the various dimensions may interact complexly with each other. To date, such basic research in the particular domain of the medical practice has not been conducted, so that the actual quantification of this schema has yet to be worked out. However, the principle is quite straightforward, and can be unequivocally illustrated, at least at the extreme ends of the dimension. For instance, a working-class female will be at a greater distance culturally from her middle-class male doctor, than say a male dentist or chemist.

The second hypothesis states that the greater the cultural gap between doctors and their patients, the less effectively will they be able to communicate with each other. This hypothesis is likely to be strenuously denied by most doctors, who in all sincerity believe that they treat all their patients equally. The doctors will maintain that they give exactly the same professional service to working-class patients as they do to the upper- or middle-classes, and have no difficulty in making themselves understood with the vast majority of their patients irrespective of their sex and ethnic or class origins. This denial is partly due to the previously discussed hidden nature of the communication barriers that may exist between persons using the same language. Two native Englishmen talking to each other hardly expect to be misunderstood, and will not notice that they are at cross-purposes except under the more acute conditions of non-correspondence in meaning. Clearly, this can be a potentially dangerous situation in a medical consultation. If either the doctor or the patient has been misunderstood, but neither becomes aware that they are at cross-purposes, the management of the patient's illness may be hampered.

What evidence is there for these propositions? Recently, David Pendleton and I (Pendleton and Bochner, 1980) conducted a study to test the hypothesis that the cultural gap between doctors and their patients has a detectable and potentially restricting effect on their communication patterns. In the study, cultural distance was defined in terms of differences in social class; and the criterion of communication effectiveness was the amount and quality of medical information that the doctors conveyed to their various patients. The study will now be described in greater detail.

9 COMMUNICATION PATTERNS AS A FUNCTION OF SOCIAL CLASS SIMILARITY-DISSIMILARITY

Seventy-nine routine general practice consultations were videotaped. Six doctors participated in the study, and all were middle-class males, with practices in the Thames Valley.

The patients were all adult whites, ranging in age from 16 to 79, and included 34 males and 45 females. The patients knew that they were being videotaped, having given their prior consent, but the taping did not appear to have any effect on the behaviour of either the patients or the doctors. Great care was taken with placing the video recording equipment so that it was quite unobtrusive, and both doctors and patients seemed to ignore the presence of the camera.

The patients were divided into three groups according to their socio-economic-status (SES). This classification resulted in 20 patients (15 males and five females) being categorized as low, 20 (six males and 14 females) as medium, and 39 patients (13 males and 26 females) as high social class members.

Two judges independently rated each videotaped consultation. Five measures were taken: (1) The *duration* of each consultation; (2) The number of statements in which the doctor *volunteered* health-related *information*; (3) The number of statements in which the doctor *volunteered* a health-related *explanation*; (4) The number of statements in which the doctor gave health-related *information* in answer to a *question*; and (5) The number of statements in which the doctor gave a health-related *explanation* in answer to a *question*. Thus, only statements with medical content were included in the tally. Re-assurance and directions regarding medication were excluded, unless an explanation was involved. On the infrequent occasion when there was a discrepancy between the two raters, that tape was played again, and the difference resolved by negotiation.

The data were analysed to test the hypothesis that culture distance between doctor and patient will affect the quantity and quality of information exchange taking place. Specifically, the hypothesis implies that higher SES patients will have longer consultations; and request and receive more medically related information and explanation, than lower SES patients.

The rather complex analysis is presented in full in the original report (Pendleton and Bochner, 1980). The results confirmed all the hypotheses: The average length of the consultations in the low, medium and high conditions was 5·26, 6·31 and 7·31 minutes respectively. The mean number of volunteered information units per consultation was 1·60, 2·40 and 3·15 respectively. The mean number of volunteered explanation units was 1·10, 1·20 and 2·10. The mean number of information units in response to a question was 0·70, 1·55 and 2·46. Finally, the mean number of explanations per consultation in response to a question was 0·25, 0·80 and 1·10 respectively.

The alternative explanation was considered that the pattern in the data could be the result of higher SES patients bringing more complex medical problems to the doctor, requiring greater treatment time and more information exchange. To check on this possibility, a diagnosis was obtained from the doctors for each patient, and the consultations were classified into *simple* (one physical problem only) or *complex* (more than one physical problem, and/or a psychosomatic problem). No differences were found between the three SES groups in the proportion of simple to complex problems, thereby ruling out the likelihood that the results were being confounded by a systematic positive relationship between SES and illness complexity. The data therefore support the conclusion that culture distance acts as a barrier to effective communication in medical settings.

The data were further inspected qualitatively for clues as to the dynamics underlying the obtained results. Pendleton and I spent 40 hours each, viewing the tapes. It soon became obvious to us that the doctors were not deliberately discriminating against their working-class patients. However, what also became clear was that the doctors were more comfortable and less formal with patients from their own sub-culture. Similarly, upper-class patients were more confident, talked and listened more, and asked more questions. In effect, they fitted better into the role of the patient, *as defined by the doctor*, than did working-class patients.

Cartwright (1964) has suggested that doctors interpret the diffidence of working-class patients to mean that these individuals do not want to know about their medical condition. We have no direct data on the attributions that the doctors in the study made about their "silent" patients. However, there was nothing in the tapes to indicate that the physicians made the assumption that working-class patients are not curious about their condition. But there were several hints that any diffidence and awkwardness that occurred on either side, was due to the social distance and status imbalance of the doctor and the patient.

10 CONCLUSION

The empirical study indicates that communication difficulties in medical settings bear a remarkable resemblance to communication difficulties in cross-cultural settings. There is support, therefore, for the idea that the cross-cultural/social skills model may provide the base for a new and useful approach to the analysis and enhancement of doctor–patient communication.

In practical terms, the model implies that communication effectiveness depends on the doctors becoming more sensitive to the frames of reference, linguistic usage, and life styles of the patients. In the taped consultations referred to earlier, most doctors probably assumed that the patients fully participated in the culture of the consulting room, meaning that the patients knew, understood and accepted the rules regulating the encounter, rules incidentally which were made by the doctor. The assumption that the patients fully entered into the consulting room culture was not always sustained, meaning that not all patients understood what they were expected to do or how they were expected to behave; nor did all patients freely agree with the implicit or explicit demands of the doctor. The data suggest that the discrepancy between "ideal" and actual patient behaviour increased as their socio-economic-status decreased, but in one sense very few individuals enacted with any great skill the social role of the patient, irrespective of their class standing. Support for this assertion is based on the low absolute level of information exchange evident in all three groups of patients. Although the upper-class patients asked for and received significantly more information than the others, even so in absolute terms they were apparently remarkably uninquisitive about their medical condition. This is contrary to anecodotal evidence that many patients complain about not receiving sufficient information from doctors, evidence that is supported by studies showing that patients are interested in finding out as much as possible about their illness (Cartwright, 1967; Ley and Spelman, 1967). The present study suggests that patients seem to be inhibited from asking for such information at a time when it would be most appropriate—during the consultation. Why is this so?

The most likely explanation is that many patients lack the social skills necessary to make such a request without feeling embarrassed or somehow unreasonable. The inability of some patients to ask the right question in the right way at the right time, is paralleled by the inability of many doctors to convey the culture of the consulting room to their patients. In the tapes, the doctor seldom began the consultation by saying, in effect: "Look, this is what I expect you to do and say, this is what I intend to do, these are the aims we hope to achieve". All this was left largely implicit, and the degree to which different patients "correctly" responded to the situation varied substantially. In general, those patients having a greater cultural affinity with their doctors, tended to be less confused about their roles than those more distant from the ethos of the medical profession and its middle-class assumptions.

In summary, the medical consultation, like any stylized social encounter, has a set of rules and assumptions, a culture. These rules and assumptions are better known by some groups than by others. They are probably best known by the doctor and people similar to the doctor, and least well known by people dissimilar to the doctor. Furthermore, the medical consultation, like any stylized social encounter, can be thought of as a mutually sustaining or inhibiting sequence of actions and reactions. Social episodes can either proceed smoothly, or falter and limp along, depending on the social skills of the participants in maintaining the interaction. Encounters are likely to be successful if the participants respond to each other appropriately; know when to speak and when to remain silent, when to express and when to inhibit their feelings; and emit and correctly interpret the appropriate non-verbal signals of posture, gesture and eye gaze. Some persons are better equipped than others successfully to negotiate a medical consultation. Presumably the most skilled are the doctors themselves, partly because they make the rules in the first place; and people similar to the doctor are more likely to possess the requisite social skills than culturally dissimilar individuals.

Certain implications follow from viewing the doctor–patient relationship in terms of culture similarity–dissimilarity. To improve communication effectiveness in the general practice consultation, the model suggests that doctors could adopt the role of culture trainers, teaching the culture of the medical consultation to those of their patients lacking the appropriate knowledge and skills. In effect this would mean explicitly telling the patients what was expected of them, and teaching them the behaviours inherent in the role of the medical patient. Modelling and encouraging the desired behaviour would be central to the success of such a training programme, since learning at the intellectual or cognitive level does not necessarily translate into the practical domain of action. Children do not learn to swim in the classroom, but in the pool. Likewise, merely telling patients, for example, that they should ask for more information, is not sufficient. Such a request will probably only result in an embarrassed silence, because the patient, although now aware that it is appropriate to ask questions, may not know what questions to ask, and how to make these requests. The doctor has to model the required behaviour, give examples, and take the patient through the actual paces of requesting and receiving health-related information. Such learning is unlikely to be instantaneous. Rather, it will take place over several consultations, be cumulative in its effect, and succeed best if it is conducted within a climate of mutual trust and openness. As the cultures of the doctor and the patient draw closer, the quality, quantity, and effectiveness of their communications ought to improve, leading not just to better medical care, but to greater job satisfaction for the doctor.

REFERENCES

Argyle, M. (1982). Inter-cultural communication. In *Cultures in Contact: Studies in Cross-cultural Interaction* (S. Bochner, ed.). Pergamon Press, Oxford.
Argyle, M., Furnham, A. and Graham, J. G. (eds) (1981). *Social Situations*. Cambridge University Press, Cambridge.
Bochner, S. (1982). The social psychology of cross-cultural relations. In *Cultures in Contact: Studies in Cross-cultural Interaction* (S. Bochner, ed.). Pergamon Press, Oxford.
Bochner, S. (in preparation). *The Psychology of the Dentist–Patient Relationship.*
Bochner, S. and Wicks, P. (eds) (1972). *Overseas Students in Australia.* The New South Wales University Press, Sydney.
Brislin, R. W. and Pedersen, P. (1976). *Cross-cultural Orientation Programs.* New York: Gardner Press, New York.
Cartwright, A. (1964). *Human Relations and Hospital Care.* Routledge and Kegan Paul, London.
Cartwright, A. (1967). *Patients and their Doctors.* Routledge and Kegan Paul, London.
Collett, P. (1982). Meetings and misunderstandings. In *Cultures in Contact: Studies in Cross-cultural Interaction* (S. Bochner, ed.). Pergamon Press, Oxford.
Furnham, A. and Bochner, S. (1982). Social difficulty in a foreign culture: An empirical analysis of culture shock. In *Cultures in Contact: Studies in Cross-cultural Interaction* (S. Bochner, ed.). Pergamon Press, Oxford.
Harré, R. (1977). The ethogenic approach: theory and practice. In *Advances in Experimental Social Psychology. Volume 10* (L. Berkowitz, ed.). Academic Press. New York.
Levine, R. V., West, L. J. and Reis, H. T. (1980). Perceptions of time and punctuality in the United States and Brazil. *J. Personal. Soc. Psychol.* **38**, 541–550.
Ley, P. and Spelman, M. S. (1967). *Communicating with the Patient.* Staples, London.
Pendleton, D. A. (1981). A situational analysis of general practice consultations. In *Social Situations* (M. Argyle, A. Furnham and J. G. Graham, eds). Cambridge University Press, Cambridge.
Pendleton, D. A. and Bochner, S. (1980). The communication of medical information in general practice consultations as a function of patients' social class. *Soc. Sci. Med.* **14A**, 669–673.
Royal College of General Practitioners (1972). *The Future General Practitioner.* Royal College of General Practitioners, London.
Secord, P. F. and Backman, C. W. (1964). *Social Psychology.* McGraw-Hill, New York.
Triandis, H. C. (1975). Culture training, cognitive complexity and interpersonal attitudes. In *Cross-cultural Perspectives on Learning* (R. W. Brislin, S. Bochner, and W. J. Lonner, eds). Wiley/Halstead, New York.

7 The Consultation: A Social Psychological Analysis

Joseph Jaspars, Jennifer King and David Pendleton

1 INTRODUCTION

One of the aims of medical treatment in general practice consultations is, where appropriate, to reduce a patient's concern about the problems presented. A dissatisfied patient who is still worried when he or she leaves the surgery, is less likely to comply with the doctor's recommendations. It has been shown that one of the reasons why sound medical advice very often does not have the intended effect is simply that the patient does not do what the doctor tells him to do (see Chapter 4, this volume). Understanding patient compliance is therefore of considerable importance for improving health care. Many factors have been shown to affect this specific form of health behaviour (Becker and Maiman, 1975). The Health Belief Model proposed by Rosenstock (1966) suggests that compliance depends upon specific beliefs held by the patient about the illness and advice in question (see Chapter 5, this volume). It seems obvious that the doctor is in a unique position to influence the patient's concern or feeling of threat and that, if he fails to give the patient confidence and reassurance in addition to effective medical treatment, the patient will be dissatisfied and will be less likely to comply with the doctor's advice. If we want to achieve a better understanding of the effect of medical treatment, it seems we have to pay more attention to certain social and psychological aspects of the consultation. This chapter analyses the consultation in terms of a two-way process of social influence. Communication difficulties are examined from the viewpoint of both doctor and patient, as well as the aspects of communication which relate to the patient's reduction in concern. Finally, we attempt to go beyond simply the communication process, to an examination of a particular aspect of patients' health beliefs. This section discusses the potential influence of patients' causal attributions or "lay explanations" of illness which, it is argued, potentially affect their readiness to comply with medical advice.

Section 2 begins, therefore, with an analysis of the two-stage "reciprocal influence" process of the consultation. Unless each "phase" of the communication occurs successfully from the viewpoint of both doctor and patient, communication difficulties will arise. Section 3 considers the sources of these communication difficulties, as seen by the doctor. Section 4, on the other hand, considers the patients' judgements of good or bad consultations. Section 5 looks at factors which significantly reduce patients' concern, and the effectiveness of persuasive communication by the doctor. Finally, Section 6 introduces two important social psychological theories as frames of reference for discussing "lay explanations" of illness and the concept of "control" over one's health. In conclusion, we argue that a synthesis of these various social psychological notions can significantly increase our understanding of the communication process in the consultation, by providing a sound theoretical framework.

2 THE CONSULTATION AS A SOCIAL INFLUENCE PROCESS

To some extent the behaviour of doctor and patient is determined by the role each of them plays in the encounter. As in any functional or task orientated encounter, social and emotional influences might also play an important role. If communication problems arise between doctor and patient, the doctor is simply not in a position to accomplish his task effectively. It may even prevent him from arriving at a diagnosis. But this is only one side of the communication process in which the patient acts as sender and the doctor as receiver. Doctor–patient communication also implies that the doctor should act as communicator (sender) and the patient as receiver. This is an added component in the interaction process, since the doctor not only wants to transmit information to the patient about his illness, but also has to convince or persuade the patient to follow a particular course of action. In short, one social-psychological aspect of the communication involves attempts by the doctor to *change* the belief or concern of the patient.

The communication phase, in which the patient *informs* the doctor about his health or problems, is essentially similar to the phase we have just described. It is not sufficient for the patient to present information to the doctor in a clear and unambiguous way. He must also be sure that the doctor pays *attention* to the complaint, *understands* the information and takes the complaint *seriously* enough to take action. In other words, no change in beliefs or behaviour on the part of either the doctor or the patient is expected to take place, if the communication breaks down in any of the phases of the persuasive communication process. We are therefore dealing with a two-stage process of reciprocal influence, in which doctor and patient influence each other. We can summarize this schematically (see Fig. 7.1) in line with the suggestions made by Pendleton in Chapter 1.

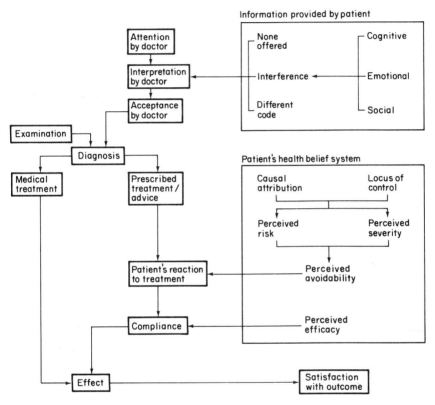

Fig. 7.1. Schematic representation of the two-stage, reciprocal social influence process in the consultation.

Figure 1 illustrates the three major aspects of doctor–patient communication which we have studied. The information provided by the patient can seem distorted in various ways preventing the doctor from fully understanding the patient's complaint. The diagram also represents the various components of the consultation which broadly falls into two stages or phases. The first stage is the intake or input phase which leads to the diagnosis. Secondly, there is the output phase which leads to the management of the problem and specific recommendations by the doctor. It is at the output stage that the patient's beliefs play a major role. Each of these three aspects of the consultation process will now be considered in detail.

3 DOCTOR–PATIENT COMMUNICATION: DIFFICULTIES REPORTED BY DOCTORS

In a previous study (Pendleton, Jaspars and Tate, unpublished) communication difficulties experienced by 23 doctors in 920 general practice consultations have been reported. The results obtained in this study were based upon questionnaires completed immediately after each of the first ten consultations on four pre-specified days. The answer to the various questions have been analysed in various ways (see Pendleton *et al.*), but here we are concerned only with the answers given by the doctors to the open-ended question "Were there any problems of communication?" It turned out that the doctors reported communication difficulties in 206 consultations out of the total of 920 (22%). The types of communication difficulties reported in these 206 consultations were content—analysed by three independent judges, who placed the answers into any one of the 32 categories. Inter-judge reliability appeared to be satisfactory (Kendall's $W = 0.73$). The answers were subsequently classified into a number of higher order categories, which were devised to represent the major components of the communication process. The first distinction to be made is between difficulties experienced by the doctor in communicating to the patient, and the difficulties experienced by the doctor, in the communication from the patient. The first category represents far fewer difficulties than the latter (13·5% vs 79%; 7·5% were not classifiable). This result may indicate simply a bias on the part of the doctor, since the former difficulties are more likely to reflect upon the doctor's competence, whereas the latter seem to reflect some difficulty of communication on the part of the patient. We will return to this point when we discuss the patients' views about good and bad consultations. The difficulties reported by the doctor in communicating to the patient seemed to be largely in the field of persuasive communication aimed at changing the patient's beliefs or attitudes. In 37% of these cases (18 out of 49) the doctor mentioned that he was unable to influence the patient or persuade him that there was (or was not) a problem. This difficulty was attributed by the doctor to a few different causes. Most often it appeared to the doctor that the patient did not believe him or had no confidence in him (39% of these difficulties) and somewhat less because the patient did not appear to understand the doctor (14%). Occasionally patient and doctor appeared to be at cross purposes (10%). The apparent psychological reactions of the patient to the communication by the doctor thus seem to lie mainly in one or two of the major components of the attitude change process. The doctors did not report that the patients failed to pay attention to their advice. Rather, the difficulties appeared to occur more often in the second phase of the change process. That is, although the patient in general understood the doctor, he was not persuaded by the advice or information.

Let us now consider the problems reported about the communication from the patient to the doctor. Here we see a completely different structure compared with the one we have first discussed. The problems seem to fit much more a general information theory concerning the nature of the *channel* used and the "noise" which appears to occur in the information transmission process. The first and obvious (though infrequent) difficulty, appears to be that the patient communicates very little or not at all (11% of the difficulties), either because he is unable to (e.g. a young child, or because of a lack of knowledge), or because he withholds information, sometimes being deliberately obstructive. Functionally equivalent to this category of difficulties are the problems which arise from the use of a "communication code" by the patient with which the doctor is unfamiliar (6% of the total 206). These difficulties appear to be mainly language problems having to do with dialect or differences in social class. Although this is a relatively rarely reported category of problems, Pendleton, Jaspars and Tate (op. cit.) and Pendleton and Bochner (1980), were able to show that the social class of the patient was quite an important predictor of communication difficulties and of whether or not the doctor would volunteer explanations to the patient.

The main category of communication difficulties between doctor and patient appears to be interference of some sort in the transmission of information (62% of the total). These interferences may be of three types: cognitive, emotional and social. *Cognitive* interference, for example, is mainly due to the fact that the patient presents more than one problem simultaneously and thus confuses the doctor. *Emotional* interference is mainly because the patient appears to be anxious, shy, depressed or nervous, but in quite a number of cases the doctor reports that he experiences an adverse reaction to the patient (bored, irritated).

The findings seem to point in the direction of a major initial obstacle for the effective treatment of the patient by the doctor. Discriminant analysis of the other responses to the same questionnaire (Pendleton, Jaspars and Tate) largely confirms the results of the content analysis of the free responses reported here. Emotional interference with the information transmission by the patient to the doctor and the social class of the patient discriminate best between consultations with and without communication difficulties. These results, however, represent only the views of the doctors. The next section therefore considers the judgements of patients about general practice consultations.

4 GOOD AND BAD CONSULTATIONS:
THE PATIENTS' VIEWS

In another study, Pendleton (unpublished) extensively interviewed 44 persons (carefully chosen to vary in age, sex and social class) about their expectations and experiences regarding consultations in general practice. The results of this study are reported more fully elsewhere, but we will consider here the answers given by the respondents to two open-ended questions. In one part of the interview the respondents were asked to think of any visit they had made to any family doctor which was particularly good or bad and to elaborate this answer by trying to formulate "what made it so good" or "what made it so bad". The answers to these two questions were subsequently categorized into six major categories corresponding to the various phases of the communication process:

(1) The attention paid by the doctor to the information presented by the patient.

(2) The interpretation or understanding of the information by the doctor.

(3) The acceptance of the information by the doctor. This category also includes the acceptance of the patient as a person.

(4) Remarks made about the medical examination itself.

(5) Observations related to the diagnosis.

(6) Comments about the prescribed or actual treatment.

There was general agreement over the features of both good and bad consultations—such that if the presence of a particular feature was seen as "good", its absence was also seen as "bad". Most remarkable perhaps, was that in both the positive and the negative cases, the respondents mention much more often psychological (72%) rather than medical (28%) factors. In the good consultation, respondents mentioned that the medical examination was quick, thorough and efficient (12%) and that the treatment was quick and effective (15%). The medical remarks about bad consultation were similar in nature: the examination was not thorough and the diagnosis was wrong (10%), or the treatment was seen as ineffective (18%).

The majority of the positive and negative remarks referred, as indicated above, to social-psychological factors in the consultation process. The predominant reply both in the negative and positive cases referred to the fact that the doctor took the patient seriously. He accepted, or did not accept, him as a person, took the complaint seriously or did not, and showed, or did not show, concern (21% in good consultations; 27% in bad consultations). Such remarks were often preceded in the interview by comments about the fact that the doctor was prompt, took his time in good consultations (16%) and showed interest and understanding (15%), whereas, in bad consultations, patients complained about the fact that the doctor did not have time for them, did not seem interested (27%) or did not seem to understand them (13%).

With respect to the second phase of the consultation, respondents rarely mentioned that the doctor did or did not explain the diagnosis (respectively 4% in good and 3% in bad consultations) but they mentioned quite often, with respect to the treatment in good consultations, that the doctor reassured them and gave them confidence. It is with respect to the treatment that the difference between good and bad consultations, as perceived by the patient, showed most clearly. When the patient felt that the treatment was ineffective, then that was apparently sufficient reason for being dissatisfied, whereas a good consultation can be positively appreciated for *two* reasons, either because the treatment was effective or because the doctor gave the patient confidence or reassurance. From further analysis it became clear that both reasons were indeed mentioned as independent causes of satisfaction with good consultations.[1]

We can summarize the results of this study in the form of a modal description of good and bad consultations as perceived by the respondents. A good consultation was one in which the treatment was effective or reassuring (29 out of the 44 people interviewed); the patient was accepted as a person, his complaints were taken seriously (20), the doctor paid prompt attention to the complaint, took his time (15) and showed understanding (14). A quick, thorough and efficient examination (11) and explanation of the diagnosis were appreciated (5). A bad consultation was one in which the doctor paid no attention (19), did not treat the patient as a person (19), prescribed the wrong treatment (14), showed no understanding (9), made the wrong diagnosis (4) and did not explain (5).

Considering the results of the two studies reported above we can see which factors specifically might be important as determinants of the psychological effects of the consultation. Apart from the patient's health beliefs (see Chapter 5, this volume) there appear to be two main "bottlenecks" in the communication process between patient and doctor. The first one is probably in the communication by the patient to the doctor, due to emotional factors on the part of either the patient or the doctor. The second appears to be the doctor's acceptance of the patient as a person and the information provided.

In order for the doctor to make a diagnosis and reduce the patient's concern it seems that it is not just "task-related" aspects that are important. The social and emotional aspects of the consultation also have a significant effect on patient satisfaction and anxiety reduction. We now turn to the last phase of the communication process.

5 THE PSYCHOLOGICAL EFFECTS OF MEDICAL TREATMENT

We have argued at the beginning of this chapter that the psychological effects of the communication from doctor to patient can be seen as the outcome of a specific social influence process in which the doctor (the "source") tries to affect a patient's (the "receiver") concern about his illness. Jaspars (1978; 1982) has argued that the results of virtually all persuasive communication studies can be understood as the outcome of a social influence process which depends on these general parameters:

(a) The change in the attitude or judgement of the receiver.

(b) The weight of the source of communication for a particular attitude of the receiver with respect to the source.

(c) The weight of the receiver's initial attitude.

(d) Attitude advocated by the source as perceived by the receiver.

(e) The initial attitude of the receiver.

In general, the change in attitude is conceived here as a function of the discrepancy in initial attitude or judgement between source and receiver and the relative weight to be assigned to the source. This general model can be applied more specifically to the case of doctor–patient communication. It can be used, in effect, to predict the relative effectiveness of the persuasive communication by the doctor. We will first discuss the design of a pilot study in which the analysis of the communication process was tested and illustrated.

In a large scale study of doctor–patient communication, Pendleton has recorded on videotape approximately 100 naturally occurring general practice consultations and also conducted interviews with doctor and patient before and after the consultation. From these recordings we selected 12 consultations (four by each of three different doctors) in which psychological and physical complaints of a serious and not serious nature occurred equally often. The behaviour of the doctor and the patient was observed by six pairs of judges who categorized the behaviour with the aid of a category scheme based upon Bales' interaction process analysis (Bales, 1950). For the purpose of the present analysis the original 12 categories of Bales have been reduced to the four main classifications of positive and negative emotional behaviour, active task behaviour (mainly asking questions and volunteering information) and reactive task behaviour (mainly providing answers by giving information, explanations and directions). The inter-rater reliability of the judgements was satisfactorily high except for the category of negative emotional behaviour on the part of the doctor which occurred too infrequently to be taken into account in the analysis.

From the interviews conducted by Pendleton, we also had information about the degree to which the doctor was concerned about the patient's illness (rating of seriousness on a five point scale) and the concern of the patient about his or her illness before and after the consultation. One would expect that in an effective consultation the doctor will be able to convey his concern to the patient so that the patient's concern will change in the direction of the view held by the doctor. We do not think that doctors will always deal well with the patients' concern or that they will necessarily want to communicate their concern to the patient. But we *do* expect that the consultation should usually be able to reduce the patient's concern. For the 12 consultations which we analysed this was true. There was a statistically significant reduction in the ratings of concern by the patients from before to after the consultations of approximately one scale point. Because we selected consultations in which both serious and non-serious cases occurred, the ratings of seriousness by the doctor and concern by the patient varied considerably and also showed a great variation in discrepancy.

With reference to our model of attitude change mentioned earlier, the next question now concerns the relative effectiveness of the persuasive communication by the doctor. The interesting finding here was that six out of seven correlations between the social behaviour of doctor and patient with the relative effectiveness of the communication were significantly negative. In other words, it appeared that, irrespective of the nature of the communication, there was less change in concern on the part of the patient the more both doctor and patient talked to each other. A likely explanation for this result is that psychological and/or serious complaints are more difficult for the doctor to deal with, which may mean that the consultation takes a relatively long time and a good deal of communication with relatively little effect. Analysis of variance of the total amount of communication showed that this was the case. Both seriousness and the psychological nature of the complaint increased significantly the total amount of communication. For this reason we subsequently analysed the relationship between the relative amount of *specific forms* of social behaviour (e.g. number of questions asked, divided by the total amount of behaviour) and the relative effectiveness of the communication. It now appeared that only one form of behaviour was significantly related to the effectiveness of the communication. If the doctor asked relatively many questions there appeared to be more relative change in the concern of the patient $(r=0.68)$.[2]

Overall, the pattern of these results seems to be fairly clear. Persuasive communication from the doctor to the patient seems to be most effective if neither the doctor nor the patient (have to) communicate extensively, but, to the extent that they do, concern is most reduced when a relatively large proportion of the interaction is taken up by the doctor asking questions. This pattern seems to occur significantly more often when the patient's complaint is not serious and of a clearly physical nature. In other words, the doctor appears to be most effective psychologically when the problem that is presented to him is one with which he can easily cope, from a medical point of view. In these cases, no extensive exchange of information is required. The doctor knows what to ask and the patient's concern is consequently reduced more. For the 12 consultations we have analysed in detail, limitation of the total amount of communication and the relative amount of asking questions does predict the effectiveness of the communication relatively well (Multiple $R = 0.77$).

First, the moderately high multiple correlation we obtained leaves 40% of the variance in effectiveness unexplained. Secondly, we have done no more than show that non-serious physical complaints are easier for the doctor not only clinically, but also when trying to reduce the patient's concern. The hard question comes when we try to understand the effectiveness of doctor–patient communication when complaints are serious and have psychological aspects. In future studies, we hope to devote special attention to these problems, but the example illustrates the technique. What is more, reduction of concern is only one possible outcome measure which we have chosen to test our social psychological model. Other outcome measures, such as the patient's compliance with the doctor's advice, may require other activities on the doctor's part. Compliance, moreover, may be incompatible with reduction in concern brought about in the way described, since this may create doctor-dependence and the lack of willingness on the patient's part to accept appropriate responsibility for their own recovery and health maintenance. Finally, we should realize that we have so far not concerned ourselves with the patients' health beliefs, their perceptions of the costs and benefits of the treatment and their attributions of the cause of the problem. It is to these issues that we shall now turn.

6 PATIENTS' BELIEFS AND EXPLANATIONS

Chapter 5 in this volume has already demonstrated that the Health Belief Model is the best theoretical approach, to date, to explain how patients' beliefs can affect health behaviour and compliance. Nevertheless, it has become apparent that the Health Belief Model, as it stands, may not be adequate to explain many types of health behaviour. It is not clear, for example whether the model can be generalized to most types of illness or health behaviours. A recent study by King and Jaspars has shown that the concepts of risk and severity are not always related to the concept of avoidability, as the Health Belief Model tends to suggest. The notion of risk differs, clearly, according to the type of illness in question, and so does the relationship between risk and prevention. This would suggest that health behaviour, or "avoidability", is governed by factors other than risk and severity. Research on the Health Belief Model has also demonstrated that perceived costs-versus-benefits of treatment is an important determinant of health behaviour. But what the model does not include are the simple "common-sense" explanations that people have about the cause of a particular illness. It does not predict when people will see an illness as caused by environmental (external) factors or personal (internal) ones. More generally, it does not predict when an illness will be seen as within a person's control or outside it—governed by some external influence. Neither is it clear what determines perceptions of risk and severity in the first place. It seems likely that causal explanations of the origins of an illness may be important antecedents of other health beliefs, and as such may also have implications for health behaviour and compliance.

The following discussion will therefore focus on two theoretical concepts, the first of which will attempt to throw some light on the subject of patients' feelings of control over their health, and the second on their common-sense causal explanations of illness. These concepts can then be combined with the existing framework of the Health Belief Model, in order to formulate a more comprehensive theory of patient health beliefs.

6.1 Patients' Locus of Control

One particular concept recently applied to the study of compliance is a personality characteristic known as "locus of control". The concept is an attempt to characterize individuals in terms of the extent to which they believe they control events. Someone with an "external" locus of control tends to be fatalistic, believing events to be determined by external forces such as chance and thus feeling powerless to influence these events. An "internal" individual believes that events are within his or her personal control.

This idea has been applied with considerable success to the area of health behaviour (Strickland, 1978). To quote just a few examples: Kirscht and Rosenstock (1977) found that lower levels of adherence to an antihypertensive regimen were associated with a lesser sense of personal control and a greater dependence on the doctor. Becker and colleagues (1977) found that greater feelings of control over life in general, and health matters in particular, were related to better compliance with dietary instructions, with medication regimens and with recommendations to obtain preventive health services for children. A study by Pennebaker *et al.* (1977) suggests that lack of control can lead to increased reporting of physical symptoms. The locus of control principle has also been frequently applied in the study of smoking. Research has found (James *et al.*, 1965) that non-smokers are more likely to be "internal" than smokers. "Internals" tend also to be able to change their smoking habits to a greater extent than "externals". Research into birth control has produced similar kinds of findings (MacDonald, 1970)—more "internals" report practising contraception than do "externals". Finally, internal locus of control has also been related to other preventive behaviours such as seat belt use and preventive dental care (Williams, 1972) and inoculations (Dabbs and Kirscht, 1971).

It appears, then, that "internals" seem more likely to engage in positive health behaviour and these findings have implications for doctor–patient communication, particularly for improving compliance with medical advice. Recent evidence (Best and Steffy, 1975) suggest that the type of treatment is often associated with locus of control in determining treatment outcome. This could be seen to imply that it may be useful to tailor treatment to the individual's locus of control. For example, an "internal" programme could provide more choice of treatment, more involvement of the patient in making choices, and in general, strong emphasis on individual, personal responsibility. It is not necessarily the case, however, that an internally orientated treatment is always more conducive to positive health behaviour. In some instances, evidence has indicated that it may be more functional to hold external beliefs. An "external" programme might therefore be designed to influence individuals who believe in chance, to believe that their health can be controlled, even if it is dependent on "powerful others" (i.e. the doctor). A belief that events can be controlled is preferable to the belief that fate will take its course since it will result in health maintenance. This type of treatment might also stress reliance on social support systems and the importance to the individual of complying with health professionals' advice. The significant point about both types of treatment programmes, however, is that they suggest constructive and systematic methods for encouraging the patient to adopt increasing personal responsibility for his or her own health.

The major significance of the concept of locus of control is that it is not only another type of subjective perception and thus in itself a "health belief", but rather that it can be used to explain and predict other health beliefs, namely perceived vulnerability and severity. The addition of the concept of locus of control to the Health Belief Model would considerably increase the model's predictive value.

Unfortunately, despite the advantages of invoking a concept such as locus of control to explain health behaviour, individuals are motivated by far more complex processes than simply their level of control over events. One of the most fundamental drives in human behaviour is the need to make sense of the environment. This means finding some way to explain events, and this is often achieved by searching for their causes. In the field of health and illness, this search for explanations is a common phenomenon: "How did I become ill?—what caused this disease?—why me?—why do I smoke?—why am I overweight?" and so forth. Most doctors, however, have little understanding about how their patients actually explain the causes of their illnesses. Yet these subjective explanations (as opposed to the more objective, medical ones) may be another significant determinant of health behaviour. Psychological research has investigated people's ideas about causality, under the heading of "attribution theory" which is concerned with how people "attribute" a cause to an event.

6.2 Patients' Causal Explanations of Illness

Initially, one must distinguish between "control" and "causality". An individual may believe that an illness is *caused* by something "external" such as a virus, but at the same time that the illness can be controlled by personal behaviour—in this case, being vaccinated. Conversely, a person with an external locus of control may perceive the cause of an illness as internal, such as a heart attack, but will still believe him or herself powerless to prevent another attack.

Research into attributions of causality has shown that people's explanations are often based on their attempts to serve their own best interests. This is known as a "self-serving bias". To give a specific example of how this concept has been applied to health behaviour: a study into the taking of swine flu injections showed that, first, most patients held biased beliefs that their own health was superior to that of others. Secondly, it was found, unexpectedly, that those who felt the most secure about their health were less likely to obtain the swine flu vaccination (Larwood, 1978). Presumably these patients attributed their good health internally and felt quite confident that they did not need the injection.

Another example of causal explanations about health behaviour is in studies on smoking (Eiser *et al.*, 1978). When asked to explain why they smoke, smokers often attribute the habit to an external cause such as the addictive nature of nicotine. Non-smokers, however, tend to attribute the smoking habit to some character deficit in the smoker! In this case they are making an internal attribution about the smoker. At its simplest, this is representative of the type of rationalizations made by people indulging in habits which they well know to be destructive to their health. They are, nevertheless, powerful influences on their health behaviour and their decision to comply with the preventive advice.

This is confirmed by substantial evidence in a recent review by Rodin (1978) in which she points out many important implications of patients' explanations. For example, misunderstandings between doctor and patient can often arise because each has a different view of the patient and the illness. A patient not taking his or her medication, for example, might be regarded as uncooperative by the doctor. The patient, on the other hand, might be inclined to attribute this reaction to the medicine, to the feelings of nausea induced by the drug. It is, therefore, important to the success of the treatment that the doctor attempts to understand the perspective of the patient. Conversely, if a patient has an *explanation* for an illness, which actually impairs his or her ability to cope, the doctor may provide a valuable corrective. Indeed, patients' explanations for serious illness are often based on false information leading to guilt and self-blame. For example, Taylor and Levin (1976) report that many women blame their breast cancer on premarital sex or some other guilt-provoking act. Such self-blame can either impair the ability to cope, or, on the other hand, it might actually facilitate coping, in the sense that the patient takes personal responsibility for preventing any future recurrence of the illness. In other words, preventive behaviour is strongly influenced by this type of causal explanation.

On the basis of this kind of evidence and research, there are several therapies currently developing which acknowledge the importance of modifying patients' explanations, as well as treating their physical condition. These have been applied successfully to five types of medical problems: pain (Meichenbaum, 1977); headache (Holroyd *et al.*, 1977; Reeves, 1976); "Type A" or coronary-prone behaviour (Suinn, 1977); obesity (Mahoney and Mahoney, 1976) and alcoholism (Sobell and Sobell, 1973).

Recent research has investigated, more specifically, the determinants of causal explanations, and has attempted to predict when a person will attribute an event to themselves rather than to the environment. (i.e. an internal rather than an external attribution). Kelley (1967; also see Kelley and Michela, 1979) has suggested that people use three kinds of information when making attributions for behaviour: (1) consistency-information about the degree to which an individual's behaviour has been consistent in a similar situation in the past: (2) consensus-information about the degree to which other people behave similarly in the same situation: and (3) distinctiveness-information about the degree to which an individual responds similarly to other kinds of situations. In terms of health beliefs, this kind of information may well be used when an individual is trying to explain why a particular illness occurred. Patients have many different "common-sense" explanations about different illnesses, and this is likely to affect their attitude towards treatment, preventive measures and compliance. It is also possible that these explanations may partly determine, for example, the degree of perceived risk. The probability (or risk) of catching an illness might be estimated by considering: (1) how often that person has had the illness before (consistency) (2) whether or not it is a common illness which affects many other people (consensus) and (3) whether the illness has a specific cause or several possible causes (distinctiveness).

Kelley's three types of information are not the only kinds that people use in explaining events or behaviour. According to Weiner and colleagues (1972) there are four primary factors which people use: ability, effort, task difficulty and luck. These four factors vary along the dimensions of stability and internality. Ability is viewed as a stable internal factor, while effort is viewed as an unstable internal factor. Task difficulty is considered to be a stable external factor, while luck is seen as an unstable external factor.

Although these factors have been used primarily to explain success and failure, certain correspondences with health and illness may be postulated. "Ability", being internal and stable, might be equated with genetic or metabolic factors. "Effort" would be personal health behaviour. "Task difficulty" might be the difficulty of overcoming existing stress in a job or at home, or in overcoming some other fixed environment factor. "Luck" would be the same as "fate" or the classical "external locus of control" mentioned above. Intuitively, it seems more likely that people use these types of explanations for illness than those suggested by Kelley. It is also likely, however, that explanations based on ability, effort, and so on, are themselves determined by consensus and consistency information. For example, if a child breaks a leg, his parents may consider how often this has happened before (consistency) and how many other children break their leg (consensus), before deciding whether it was just bad luck or the child's carelessness (lack of effort).

In order for these concepts to be useful they need to be integrated in some way with the existing Health Belief Model, since the relevance of this for doctor– patient communication has been established. It is suggested that a patient uses a whole array of different explanations and beliefs in his or her final decision to comply or take health measures. Although each of the factors mentioned has some part to play in this decision-making none of them is, on its own, sufficient or necessary to predict health behaviour. The sequence of the decision process can only be hypothesized, but research is in progress to investigate the types of causal explanations people make about illnesses, how these affect other health beliefs such as perceived risk and ultimately how all these factors affect health behaviour. A model has been formulated in Fig. 7.2.

7 CONCLUSIONS AND IMPLICATIONS

Figure 7.1, we have suggested, serves to summarize some of the processes thought to be at work in general practice consultations and the subsequent sections of this chapter have both elaborated its content and demonstrated research methods associated with it.

We have demonstrated that there are well documented social psychological theories which can explain some important aspects of doctor–patient communication. Certainly, the notion of a perfectly rational patient presenting

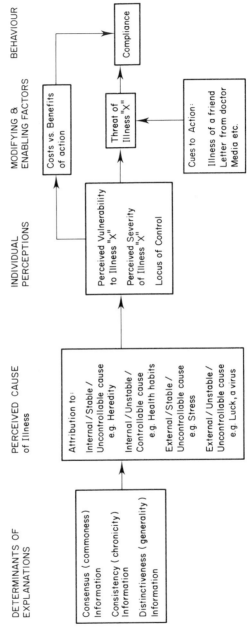

Fig. 7.2.   Proposed attribution—health belief model.

a discrete problem to a perfectly rational doctor whose training equips him to deal with all aspects of the problem will not do. First, it does not explain the findings that patients do not readily comply with the advice offered. Secondly, it does not account for the finding that doctors experience communication problems themselves in 20% of their consultations and that tension in both parties seems to be the most frequent correlate. Thirdly, it does not account for the finding that persuasion is needed, sometimes to convince the patient that they do not have any physical problem at all. Finally, it does not give us any way of understanding that patients so frequently identify a bad consultation as one in which the doctor did not take them seriously or show concern.

We are moving towards a view of the consultation process in which both doctor and patient are to be seen as possessing their own beliefs about health and illness, about their roles and about the other person. These views play their part in determining the consultation's outcomes and can influence its course just as definitely as can the nature of the complaint and the doctor's clinical expertise.

We require that consultation processes become better understood. The consultation has been, hitherto, lacking in theoretical insights and appropriate models. As a result, research in consultation processes has been piecemeal. Theory is not to be seen as the opposite of practice and, therefore, something to be avoided by all practitioners. On the contrary, theory is to be seen as the enabler of practice since an adequate theory must be able to simplify by giving order to complexity. Indeed the absence of theory is chaos, giving rise to practice based on expedience or superstition.

In the drive to understand the processes at work in the consultation, social psychological notions have a lot to say about communication. The literature on health beliefs and locus of control, moreover, can help us to explain and influence the patients' views about health and illness and, ultimately, to persuade individuals to live healthier lives. Research can then proceed from this more sound theoretical base and training can be more firmly grounded on reliable evidence rather than on doctrinaire adherence to a series of dicta.

The outcomes of medical consultations are too important to be left either to chance or to atheoretical expedience. At present, the National Health Service is spending a great deal of money providing prescriptions which are unwanted, and advice which is not followed. If, however, doctors' and patients' attempts to communicate can be aided, not only would the financial savings vindicate the effort, but the resulting increase in the satisfaction of doctor and patient, we are suggesting, would be considerable.

NOTES

1. The actual or observed probability of a respondent mentioning both

medical effectiveness and psychological confidence or reassurance is $P=0·10$, whereas the expected probability for the joint occurrence of both types of remarks is $P=0·13$.

2. There also appeared to be a significantly negative correlation with the negative socio-emotional behaviour of the doctor ($r=-0·53$), but since this behaviour hardly varied in that it was rarely present we did not include it in the present analysis.

REFERENCES

Bales, R. F. (1950). *Interaction Process Analysis: A Method for the Study of Small Groups.* Addison Wesley, Cambridge, Mass.

Becker, M. and Maiman, L. (1975). Sociobehavioural determinants of compliance with medical case recommendations. *Med. Care* 18 (1), 10–24.

Becker, M., Haefner, D., Kasl, S., Kirscht, J., Maiman, L. and Rosenstock, I. (1977). Selected psychosocial models and correlates of individual health-related behaviours. *Med. Care.* 15 (5 Suppl.), 27–46.

Best, J. and Steffy, R. (1975). Smoking modification procedures for internal and external locus of control clients. *Can. J. Behav. Sci.* 7, 155–165.

Dabbs, J. and Kirscht, J. (1971). Internal control and the taking of influenza shots. *Psych. Rep.* 28 (3), 959–962.

Eiser, J., Sutton, S. and Wober, M. (1978). Smokers' and non-smokers' attributions about smoking: a case of actor-observer differences. *Br. J. Soc. Clin. Psychol.* 17, 189–190.

Holroyd, K., Andraski, F. and Westbrook, T. (1977). Cognitive control of tension headache. *Cog. Ther. Res.* 1, 121–133.

James, W., Woodruff, A. and Werner, W. (1965). Effect of internal and external control upon changes in smoking behaviour. *J. Consult. Psychol.* 29, 184–196.

Jaspars, J. M. F. (1978). Determinants of attitudes and attitude change. In *Introducing Social Psychology* (H. Tajfel and C. Fraser, eds). Penguin Books, Harmondsworth.

Jaspars, J. M. F. (1982). Social cognition and social behaviour. In *Social Cognition and Social Behaviour* (J. Codol and J-P. Leyens, eds).

Kelley, H. (1967). Attribution theory in social psychology. *Nebraska Symposium on Motivation*, 15, 192–238.

Kelley, H. and Michela, J. L. (1979). Attribution theory and research. In *Annual Review of Psychology* (M. R. Rosenzweig and L. M. Porter, eds). Vol. 31. Annual Reviews, Palto Alto.

Kirscht, J. and Rosenstock, I. (1977). Patient adherence to antihypertensive medical regimens. *J. Comm. Hlth.* 3 (2), 115–124.

Larwood, L. (1978). Swine Flu: A field study of self-serving biases. *J. App. Soc. Psychol.* 8 (3), 283–289.

MacDonald, A. (1970). Internal-External locus of control and the practice of birth control. *Psychol. Rep.* 27, 206.

Mahoney, M. and Mahoney, K. (1976). *Permanent Weight Control.* W. W. Norton, New York.

Meichenbaum, D. (1977). *Cognitive-behaviour Modification: An Integrative Approach.* Plenum, New York.

Pendleton, D. (1982). Patients' views of general practitioners. Unpublished chapter in doctoral dissertation: University of Oxford.

Pendleton, D., Jaspars, J. M. F. and Tate, P. Doctor–patient communication: Difficulties reported by doctors. Unpublished: University of Oxford.

Pennebaker, J., Burnam, M., Schaeffer, M. and Harper, D. (1977): Lack of control as a determinant of perceived physical symptoms. *J. Pers. Soc. Psych.* **35**, 167–174.

Reeves, J. (1976). EMG-biofeedback reduction of tension headache: A cognitive skills training approach. *Biofeedback Self Regulat.* **1**, 217–225.

Rodin, J. (1978). Somatopsychics and attribution. *Pers. Soc. Psych. Bull.* **4** (4), 531–538.

Rosenstock, I. (1966). Why people use health services. *Milbank Mem. Fund Q.* **44**, 94–127.

Sobell, M. and Sobell, L. (1973). Individualized behaviour therapy for alcoholics. *Behav. Ther.* **4**, 49–72.

Strickland, B. (1978). Internal-external expectancies and health-related behaviours. *J. Consult. Clin. Psychol.* **46** (6), 1192–1211.

Suinn, R. (1977). Type A behaviour pattern. In *Behavioural Approaches to Medical treatment* (R. B. Williams and W. D. Gentry, eds). Ballinger, Cambridge.

Taylor, S. and Levin, S. (1976). The psychological impact of breast cancer. Theory and practice. In *Psychological Aspects of Breast Cancer* (A. Enelow, ed.). West Coast Cancer Foundation, San Francisco.

Weiner, B., Frieze, I., Kukla, A., Reed, I., Rest, S. and Rosenbaum, R. (1972). Perceiving the causes of success and failure. In *Attribution: Perceiving the Causes of Behaviour* (I. E. Jones, D. E. Kanouse, H. H. Kelley, R. E. Nisbett, S. Valins and B. Weiner, eds). General Learning Press, Morristown, N.J.

Williams, A. (1972a). Factors associated with seat belt use in families. *J. Saf. Res.* **4** (3), 133–138.

Williams, A. (1972b). Personality characteristics associated with preventitive dental health practices. *J. Am. Coll. Dent.* **39**, 225–234.

Part III
The Doctor–Patient Relationship

8 The Doctor–Patient Relationship in Diagnosis and Treatment

Paul Freeling

1 INTRODUCTION

The quality of communication between doctor and patient helps determine the effectiveness of the consultation in which it takes place. In order to measure the effectiveness of any act a definition of its purpose is required and the purpose may vary with the setting in which the act takes place. This chapter is concerned with consultations between patient and doctor in the setting of general practice and the ways in which the doctor–patient relationship can be used to increase their effectiveness. The medical model of diagnosis and treatment is adopted although, in the rapid and complex transactions which comprise individual consultations in general practice, these two activities are intimately inter-twined. Preventative interventions will be considered as treatments. Some of the points made in the chapter will be illustrated by a brief example drawn from a series of patient–doctor contacts.

This chapter represents a complex of beliefs and ideas rooted in the biography of its author which includes five years of what is now commonly termed "Balint training" (Balint, 1957). The notions which arose from the training-research seminars initiated at the Tavistock Clinic by the late Michael Balint now constitute the most pervasive and cohesive ideology in general practice (Stimson, 1978). This chapter is not concerned with the history of developments in the study and use of the doctor–patient relationship but sets out to describe the possibilities for its use in the here and now. These possibilities are derived both from the general purposes of providing medical care and from the characteristics of general practice as a setting for its provision.

2 THE PURPOSES OF MEDICAL CARE

The purpose of medical care is to foster health. The World Health Organisation has offered a definition of health as a state of complete physical, mental, and social well-being, not merely the absence of disease or infirmity. This ideal is seldom reached let alone maintained and a more operational definition is that "health is a satisfactory adaptation of the individual to his total environment—physical, psychological and socio-cultural" (Royal College of General Practitioners, 1972). From this statement can be derived the aim of medical care as helping each person to attain optimum development as a whole person by avoiding or correcting maladaptations or their causes.

General practitioners have a number of diverse opportunities to foster optimum development and deal with maladaptation. These arise from the provision of three types of care: first-contact care; continuing care; and preventive care. First contact care often deals with illness as yet unorganized (Balint, 1957); continuing care usually deals with illness already organized or with identified handicap; preventive care makes arrangements for doctor–patient contacts in a "no-illness situation" (Greco and Pittenger, 1966). There is of course no reason why these three types of care should not be provided at one contact: indeed the opportunistic use of first-contacts for preventive purposes has much to recommend it. Provision of these types of care, the purposes to which they are directed, and the place of general practice in the social institution medicine, have led to a number of characteristics of general practice which seem to be identifiable throughout most of the developed world.

3 THE CHARACTERISTICS OF GENERAL PRACTICE

Most of the characteristics of general practice are embodied in the following fifteen statements concerning it.
(1) Deals with undifferentiated illness and early symptomatic diagnosis;
(2) Practitioners often help patients to organize their illnesses (Balint, 1957);
(3) Is a low-technology discipline;
(4) Requires the use of estimates of probabilities and of threat in making decisions upon interventions (RCGP, 1977);
(5) Makes use of time in both diagnosis and treatment;
(6) Takes a person-centred approach to medical care (Tait, 1974);
(7) Is aware of problems of compliance, by doctors with standards of care and by patients with advice and treatment;
(8) Provides continuing care;
(9) Adopts a preventive attitude;

(10) Uses a developmental approach;
(11) Makes selective use of resources;
(12) Takes a responsibility to the community at large;
(13) Demands of its practitioners an ability to tolerate uncertainty (Thomson, 1978);
(14) Requires of its practitioners a knowledge of the functions of many other disciplines;
(15) Relies upon its practitioners having high skills in conducting interviews.

These characteristics of general practice are exhibited in, and dependent upon, the consultation between doctor–patient.

4 CHARACTERISTICS OF THE CONSULTATION IN GENERAL PRACTICE

The office (surgery) consultation in general practice has often been reported as averaging less than seven minutes (Royal College of General Practitioners, 1973). The average conceals some variation in duration, indeed it has been demonstrated (Long, 1974) that the distribution of consultation time is bimodal. Long's study indicates that GPs who have longer consultations are more flexible about the length of consultations and also have very short ones. This is related to a most important aspect of consultations derived from the continuing responsibility which is accepted by every National Health Service General Practitioner and concurred with by the patients who register with him. Continuing responsibility, which mean consultation time ignores, affords the patient the opportunity, and places upon the general practitioner an obligation, to use every consultation as part of a process, a related series of interviews (RCGP, 1972), even if each interview has, ostensibly, a different content. This responsibility has become easier to meet over the past years as a shift in emphasis has taken place away from episodic first contact care towards doctor-initiated (Morrell et al., 1970) consultations. This change reflects, presumably, a greater emphasis upon continuing and preventive care (an acceptance of responsibility for the continuing care of defined conditions, organic, psychiatric or social, and for preventive supervision such as ante-natal care, developmental assessment, cervical cytology, monitoring of contraceptive practice, or the identification of symptomless hypertension). The possibilities for person-centred medicine in the "no-illness situations" offered by these activities have been described (Greco and Pittenger, 1966). Both the management of defined conditions and the implementation of prevention usually require changes in the previous behaviour of the patient. Changes in behaviour, depend upon the effectiveness of communications made by doctor to patient just as interpretation of behaviour by the doctor depends upon making as full use as possible of all that the patient is willing to communicate.

5 VOCATIONAL TRAINING AND THE DOCTOR–PATIENT RELATIONSHIP

Management of unorganized illness is one of the tasks which distinguishes the work of the general practitioner from that of the hospital doctor. Modern programmes of vocational training are often directed, in part, towards helping the young doctor to gain skills in unravelling presentations of unorganized illness. The trainee general practitioner is expected to share with the patient the problem-solving involved using a wide range of data to do so and avoiding an artificial distinction between physical pathology and human behaviour as the cause of the malaise (Gray, 1977). The young doctor is encouraged to make his diagnoses "simultaneously in physical, psychological and social terms" (RCGP, 1972), to view psyche and soma as interactive components of the whole person rather than as alternative causes of malaise. It is easy to make treatment plans for the short-term malaise, it may be more difficult to make long-term management plans for the whole person diagnosis over a series of patient-initiated interviews, especially if the trainee is not given responsibility for continuing care (O'Flanagan, 1977; Hasler, 1978).

An understanding of the doctor–patient relationship and of its use in diagnosis and treatment will be gained more easily if the trainee is always conscious of the fact that any interaction is affected by the expectations brought to it by the participants. These expectations can originate in the perceptions each has of the other and begin with the normative beliefs each has concerning, in the case of the doctor–patient consultation, the role doctor, the role patient and interaction between these roles. They are modified over the contact or series of contacts by what each learns about the other. It is to be hoped that the result, when necessary, is to bring expectations and reality closer together. As well as normative beliefs concerning his own and the other's role, each will have expectations concerning the act sequence (Hymes, 1972) of the consultation itself. These too will be modified by experience and again it is to be hoped that the result is to bring expectations and reality closer together. The doctor's empathic responses will be based, in part, upon his perception of gaps between these two sorts of expectation and reality, together with judgements concerning the patient's flexibility of approach to bridging these gaps, of accepting the results of reality-testing.

6 EFFECTS OF COMMUNICATION AND THE DOCTOR–PATIENT RELATIONSHIP

The effect of communication is not only to impart information (informative) but also to encourage certain actions (promotive) and to produce feelings (evocative) (Browne and Freeling, 1976). A patient will be uncertain about the extent to which he or she wishes to impart information, has the ability to encourage actions by the doctor, or the right to produce feelings. The doctor must respect these uncertainties but not necessarily accept the limitations initially imposed by them. The doctor will continue to have the purpose of helping the individual to make adaptive rather than maladaptive responses. The form and content of the communications made by the patient and the effect of the doctor's communications upon the patient will depend upon the nature of the relationship between them.

The doctor–patient relationship provides the emotional environment for the consultation. The quality of the relationship affects the intellectual processes of the doctor and the patient just as the physical environment in which a lecture is given affects intelligibility through its acoustics, or attention span through its temperature and the comfort of the seats provided. The intelligibility of this chapter will be affected by the accuracy with which the wants of a reader, as yet unidentified as it is prepared, have been judged. It will be affected also by the clarity with which the material selected for presentation has been arranged. During a consultation there is feedback which enables the doctor to judge his intelligibility and the accuracy of his perceptions. The emotional environment of the consultation is affected by the degree to which the doctor seeks that feedback, shows that he seeks it, responds to it, and explains his or her response. In this way the quality of the relationship becomes part of the communication, as well as the environment for it.

There are two other important characteristics of the doctor–patient relationship. The first characteristic is that the relationship always remains, to some extent, under the control of the doctor, since he always has the opportunity of using the authority of his role, even if he uses it only at the request of the patient. This characteristic carries with it an obligation, unusual in relationships, that the doctor should try to understand how the patient uses him. His perceptions of himself and awareness of his own tendency to respond in the relationship, the doctor uses in diagnosis. His understanding of the patient's self-perception and perception of the doctor, should be used in therapy. The second characteristic the doctor–patient relationship shares with other relationships, namely that its character varies with the honesty and intimacy of what takes place within it. This characteristic is affected in a special way by the authority implicit in the doctor's role.

Intimacy is a variable which may be measurable, ranging as it does from an interaction between actors of two social roles, to a most intimate relationship between two human beings. As intimacy increases, social distance decreases: as social distance decreases, the doctor gives up the authority which is donned with the costume of the role and may be rewarded instead with the power given freely by one person to another (Freeling, 1978), based on informed trust, to offer insight to the patient. The offer of intimacy by the doctor may well be one way of pursuing the aims of optimum development and avoidance of maladaptation by the patient. It must be emphasized, however, that intimacy can be offered, but must not be demanded. A demand for intimacy backed by the authority of the doctor's role comes close to rape of the patient.

7 THE DOCTOR AS THE EQUIVALENT OF A LABORATORY INVESTIGATION

The doctor uses himself as a test instrument in several ways. He does this in part by being aware of the character of the relationship between himself and the patient. He derives this awareness by recognizing temptations to respond in a particular manner within that relationship and from his observations of the patient's behaviour. This is sometimes termed the use of empathy as a diagnostic tool and has been widely discussed in particular in terms of the value to the doctor of his feelings towards the patient (Balint and Norrell, 1973).

Two intellectual activities of the doctor which help to utilize the doctor–patient relationship in diagnosis must be highlighted. First, the doctor should identify any incongruities between components of his observations, including his empathic ones, and seek to explain them and make predictions to test his explanations. Secondly, as the relationship builds and develops, the doctor should look for consistencies and inconsistencies in the picture of it he is outlining. Consistencies act as confirmatory evidence for predictions made. Inconsistencies may lead to modifications of the picture and so to further predictions or they may be warning signs of a need for intervention. Which of these two applies, will depend upon whether or not the doctor's prediction was of maladaptive or adaptive response: that optimal or less than optimal development was likely.

The description which follows of a related series of interviews with Mrs Amy Gale will help clarify some of the points made so far.

Amy Gale is a 73-year-old widow. She and the doctor first met in October 1977, some months after the doctor joined the group of G.P.s to whose care she had been transferred 18 months earlier, when her previous G.P. retired. She had asked for a repeat prescription. The doctor, because of a distaste for giving out slips of paper to patients he had never seen, asked her to make an appointment. He was aware of the risks inherent in interfering in a "peaceful" repeat prescription and of the meanings which might be attached to its having been established (Balint *et al.*, 1970).

Mrs Gale's notes went back to 1952, when she was 47-years-old. She had had few attendances till 1956 when she was treated for hot flushes. She had been a regular attender for treatment of mild hypertension since 1968. She had been treated for joint pain since 1976, first with modern and powerful anti-inflammatory drugs which have frequent gastro-intestinal complications, and later with paracetamol.

Mrs Gale is always well-turned out. She has thick, dark hair only speckled with grey and she always smiles a lot. At the first consultation in 1977, the doctor described to her his reluctance to prescribe without consultation. She smiled sweetly and agreed to his taking her blood pressure. He asked how her joint pains were. "Oh, not so bad, doctor". Her face had changed for a moment and the doctor pursued his questions more directly. Her ankle joints and wrists were warm and puffy indicating active joint disease requiring treatment. She continued to smile and say that the pain was "not too bad". She agreed, with a smile, to some blood tests. She had an ESR of 50 and a positive serology for rheumatoid arthritis confirming the clinical impression of active disease. She remained reluctant to admit to pain, although she continued to consume paracetamol regularly. She was reluctant to try any other medicines, since such treatment had always upset her stomach in the past. She agreed with the doctor that he would keep an eye on her joints, but not insist on new treatment.

The relationship between doctor and patient at that point could be described as fairly formal, although Mrs Gale did not conform completely to the role of patient. She seemed reluctant to be seen to complain, to bother the doctor. She was, within reason, acquiescent. She seemed most concerned to present herself well, in behaviour and in appearance. She seemed to see doctors as being people who would not approve of people who complained to them. The doctor felt strongly that it was approval, even admiration that she sought, rather than affection or liking, or even treatment for her pain. The doctor suspected that her hypertension did not need treatment whilst her rheumatoid arthritis did. Management plans for these were relatively easy to formulate. His plan for the whole person was to provide the approval or admiration Mrs Gale seemed to require. This was easy, because the doctor genuinely felt these two emotions. The doctor decided not to enforce intimacy, but to use their regular meetings for very gentle probing. He noted the incongruity between denial of pain and the regular taking of pain killers, together with the results of his examination and tests. The doctor wondered if his guess as to her need for approval and admiration would be confirmed by consistencies. He assumed that Mrs Gale's wish for these was a response to some set of events in her past life. The response seemed to have been adaptive originally, but was now generalizing itself to a degree that might be maladaptive.

The doctor and Mrs Gale consulted ten more times in the next year. All consultations were, like the first one, doctor-initiated. In the event, Mrs Gale's blood pressure proved not to need treatment and her rheumatoid arthritis became quiescent without treatment. The doctor learnt that she had a married son living in Southern Ireland, a married daughter living nearby, who had a 4-year-old girl and another on the way. She had had a third child, her eldest, who died in the 1940s of miliary tuberculosis. She had been widowed twelve years ago and had no money worries. She led a reasonably active social life, which included considerable time spent helping others physically less fortunate than herself. She remained really remarkably young and fit looking and despite being herself 73 years old, Mrs Gale acted as secretary for a local community group of middle-aged people who had formed themselves in order to help elderly people. The relationship remained fairly formal, but intimate enough for both their needs. Mrs Gale's behaviour remained consistent. The doctor felt that she continued to need approval and admiration and he continued to provide it. The doctor was still uncertain as to whether her need was maladaptive or not.

Circumstances conspired for the doctor to miss seeing Mrs Gale for a couple of months and they met again in mid-March.

Mrs Gale looked her usual self and had her usual smile. The doctor asked how she was and that odd look he had noticed at their first meeting flashed across her face, a look of fleeting uncertainty. The doctor encouraged Mrs Gale to talk. She had begun to "feel rotten" quite suddenly 10 days earlier. The doctor could determine no localizing symptoms or indications of cause, and he said that he was puzzled. That look flashed across her face again. "Could it be because I'm upset doctor?" Mrs Gale said, hesitantly. The doctor encouraged her to enlarge upon this idea, knowing that doing so would increase the intimacy level of their relationship, but prepared to take the risk.

This abbreviated description of a series of twelve interviews serves to illustrate a number of points already made. It is based upon doctor-initiated contacts. It shows the formulation of diagnoses simultaneously in physical, psychological and social terms and illustrates the use of incongruities and the building up of consistencies. The description is halted at a point when an inconsistency seems to have manifested itself and the doctor has chosen to encourage an increased intimacy, a decrease in social distance, in order to examine it. If the model diagnosis followed by treatment is applied then the description stops at the point when a diagnosis is about to be formulated, the question is to be put as to whether or not Mrs Gale's preferences for a particular kind of relationship are adaptive or maladaptive. At this point it seems sensible to review the opportunities for the doctor to act as a drug (Balint, 1957) within the doctor–patient relationship.

8 THE DOCTOR AS A THERAPEUTIC AGENT

There are four broad categories of purpose to which therapy can be directed. These are:
(i) Symptom-removal;
(ii) Alteration of mechanisms linking symptoms and cause;
(iii) Removal of cause including correction of deficiency or surfeit;
(iv) Placebo effect.
Physical examples are obvious. Symptom-removal is exemplified by aspirin for headache; removal of cause by penicillin for lobar pneumonia; correction of deficiency by thyroxine for hypothyroidism; and alteration of mechanisms by steroid therapy for asthma.

The same drug can be used for different purposes in different diseases, so that aspirin besides being a symptom-remover, is also an anti-inflammatory agent, breaking the link between cause and symptoms in rheumatoid arthritis.

The right of a doctor to intervene for the purposes of avoiding maladaptive response needs to be justified. When a response is satisfactory for its intentions, it can only be termed maladaptive if it is unacceptable to society at large. The matter of whether or not deviance is illness, or a medical matter at all, will not be discussed in this chapter. When, however, a maladaptive response becomes a matter of concern to the patient, who sees it as a symptom beyond his or her control and presents it to a doctor, then it seems self-evident that it becomes a medical matter, although not necessarily one which should be organized into and labelled as disease. When there are "repetitive maladaptive behaviour patterns and attitudes to such a degree that effective functioning is impaired" (Pardes, 1977) there is, by one definition a character disorder and if this is presented to a doctor, he has a responsibility to help his patient, again without necessarily organizing it or labelling it as disease. Mrs Gale had shown a consistent behaviour pattern which the doctor identified as needing approval and admiration. It had proven maladaptive only in leading her not to complain to the doctor about pains and not to seek monitoring of a condition for which she accepted treatment. Let us return to the mid-March consultation which was left at a point when the doctor had risked increasing the intimacy of his relationship with Mrs Gale and was about to test whether or not her maladaptive response might have become more generalized so as to interfere with her effective functioning. The doctor was doing this whilst bearing in mind that sudden ill-defined malaise in a person of Mrs Gale's age, could be the first indication of sinister physical processes. The doctor had no clue as to what these processes might be and was willing to wait a short while to see what manifested itself.

In response to his invitation to talk more intimately, Mrs Gale told the doctor that her daughter's pregnancy was now hypertensive and that Mrs Gale had been tiring herself out looking after her grandchildren whilst her daughter rested. Now her daughter was to have a caesarean section if not spontaneously delivered within the week. The doctor wondered if Mrs Gale was worried that she would not be able to look after her grandchild. When asked, Mrs Gale assured him that there would be no problems: all had been arranged. That look of uncertainty crossed her face again. "What is it then?" asked the doctor. She took a deep breath and said, "It's this acquaintance I shop for," she stopped. Both doctor and Mrs Gale were silent. Mrs Gale seemed unable to continue. The doctor decided to take the plunge and risk the intimacy of presenting Mrs Gale with his perception of her then. There can be no more intimate act. "Mrs Gale," he said "It has always seemed to me that you prefer not to complain". Mrs Gale looked as if she might cry: the smile had completely gone. The doctor commented on this. Mrs Gale poured out a story about an acquaintance for whom she shopped every day, who always complained and questioned the cost of things and said that Mrs Gale had bought the wrong items and sometimes made her take them back to the shop. "Normally I can cope with her, and what she makes me do, although I don't like her," said Mrs Gale, "but not when I'm so worried about my daughter. What am I to do doctor?"

What Mrs Gale should do seemed self-evident—she should stop helping her friend, at least for the moment. It was equally obvious she could not bring herself to do so. How could the doctor best help Mrs Gale?

The distinction between authority and power was drawn earlier in this chapter. The degree of intimacy between the doctor and Mrs Gale had been increased by what Mrs Gale had just revealed about herself, that she could not cope with the behaviour of an acquaintance whom she could normally tolerate although never emulate. There still remained a considerable social distance between the doctor and Mrs Gale. The doctor had no idea how Mrs Gale had acquired her need to have approval and admiration. To explore the origin of a piece of consistent behaviour which seemed to have served Mrs Gale very well risked her ceasing to exhibit it. All human beings have behaviours some of which can be classified as "secret", others as "hidden" (Freeling, 1976). Secret behaviours are those of which people are aware but of which they are, for some reason, ashamed and so keep them, as far as possible, concealed. Hidden behaviours are hidden from the awareness of the individual concerned but can be observed by others. The doctor's statement that Mrs Gale seemed to prefer not to complain had been made without knowing whether this was a secret or a hidden behaviour, or one of which she was proud. Any further examination of that behaviour in an attempt to remove the cause would threaten to uncover a secret or discover to Mrs Gale something at present hidden from her. Even if the exploration and its findings proved acceptable to Mrs Gale it might not prove beneficial. Mrs Gale's unwillingness to complain and her eagerness to help others who did complain helped her to fill her life. She was entitled to continue to do so. There was no reason why her present predicament (Taylor, 1979) should be allowed permanently to alter her way of life.

The doctor determined to help Mrs Gale in what was, for her, a near break-down in an aspect of social functioning, by using the authority of his role to excuse her from the responsibilities she normally accepted. He pulled himself upright in his chair and said, as firmly as he could "Mrs Gale, as your doctor, I must tell you for the sake of your health to stop doing other people's shopping until you feel better in yourself. Come and see me in ten days time, after your daughter has had her baby and we'll see how you are getting on". Mrs Gale thanked him profusely, saying that she had hoped that this was what he would tell her, since she felt so ill.

The whole story is open to multiple interpretations and the doctor's actions are open to criticism. When his decisions were taken he needed to tolerate considerable uncertainty concerning the possible co-existence of serious physical disease as well as the outcome of his chosen intervention. Nevertheless the case history illustrates the use of the doctor–patient relationship in diagnosis and treatment, the treatment lying in the category of interfering with the mechanisms linking symptom and cause. It illustrates also the use of variations in intimacy and demonstrates the use of authority from the role doctor in treatment when the diagnosis had been reached via the power of intimacy. It may illustrate, also that the doctor was concerned to allow Mrs Gale to retain her personal autonomy (Stimson, 1978) and that she saw herself as having done so since she told the doctor he had done what she had hoped for.

The use of the doctor–patient relationship has been dealt with in the context of recognition and treatment of a maladaptive response which might have become, later in that relationship, a cause of malaise. In the last part of this chapter possible uses of the doctor–patient relationship will be covered in the treatment or prevention of two, more clearly defined, behavioural threats to optimum functioning. These are anxiety and depression which are two sets of response which tend to be identified as symptoms by patients.

9 THE RELATIONSHIP AS TREATMENT FOR ANXIETY

In this section treatment of the patient's perceived anxiety will be covered— although all doctors know that they sometimes use the doctor–patient relationship to reduce their own anxiety. If the prescription rate of drugs designed to reduce anxiety is a satisfactory indicator (Marks, 1978), general practitioners see many patients who complain of anxiety. There are many possible causes of anxiety and almost as many psychological theories to describe its origins. It is sometimes helpful to both doctor and patient if the source of the symptoms of anxiety is sought within the framework of stress produced by conflicts arising from incompatible goals (Tallent, 1978). Whatever the underlying reasons for the judgements made of the goals, people are often faced with decisions, the perceived outcomes of which are in conflict. There may be desirable outcomes and undesirable outcomes. Conflict may exist because only one of two desirable outcomes can result from a decision and this would be an approach–approach conflict. Conflict may exist because only one of two undesirable outcomes can result and this would be an avoidance–avoidance conflict. Much more complex is the occasion when a patient is drawn to incompatible goals each of which has both desirable and undesirable outcomes. The resolution of all conflict is by taking a decision and there is some evidence (Festinger, 1964) that we are biased in favour of our own decisions. It is important, therefore, that a general practitioner who elicits a multiple approach–avoidance conflict as source of a patient's symptoms of anxiety utilizes a suitable doctor–patient relationship to resolve it. A consultation which has the characteristics of mutual participation (Szasz and Hollender, 1956) would seem suitable. It is one of the tasks of a general practitioner to be able to set up a doctor–patient relationship, or modify an existing one, so that its characteristics are appropriate for the patient to resolve conflict within it.

Where anxiety is produced by conflict, doctors are often tempted into treatment by placebo, by telling the patient, with all the authority they possess, that there is nothing to worry about. They may be tempted into symptom-removal by treatment with benzodiazepines or they may, more properly, attempt removal of cause by the use of counselling techniques, to bring the patient to resolution of the conflict. The character of the doctor–patient relationship is obviously affected towards an increase in intimacy when a counselling style is adopted. It would seem that the relationship is pushed also towards termination, because counselling is an attempt to give autonomy back to the patient and follow-up would be inappropriate. The doctor is placed, thus, in a dilemma when the next in the process of interviews occurs for a different cause. When counselling fails, or anxiety persists after the resolution of conflict, then the doctor should assume that he was not in fact removing cause, but interfering in mechanisms which link cause and symptom. That is to say that defence mechanisms in the patient were involved in producing both the anxiety and the conflict. The doctor–patient relationship remains available as both environment and instrument for uncovering these defence mechanisms.

10 THE RELATIONSHIP AS TREATMENT FOR DEPRESSION

Until recently there was no validated causal model for depression. One hypothesis is that depression is the cardinal sign that an individual feels the equilibrium of his or her maturity to be threatened (Browne and Freeling, 1976). Maturation is seen as the ability to integrate new experiences in such a way as to produce the optimum response. Emotional immaturity is, therefore, one factor in producing the depressive reaction. There are four classes of situation which constitute threats. The first is the failure of a situation to develop in the way that one has come to expect from past experience, so that a habitual reaction is no longer appropriate; the second arises from the effects of prolonged stress, often appearing after its removal; the third class is situations giving rise to chronic frustration, when the expression of anger is inhibited; and the fourth is in situations of chronic boredom and stimulus hunger.

This hypothesis of depression as reaction to situations which threaten self-perceived maturity is erected partly on a basis of theory and partly on identification of the kinds of therapeutic activity doctors find themselves able to undertake within the doctor–patient relationship. These therapeutic activities included, acting as a confidant with whom the failure of situations to develop could be shared, and acting as a model for new coping behaviours. They included allowing the patient to work through stressful events in the safe house of a secure doctor–patient relationship; also included was the opportunity to obtain stimulus within it. As far as immaturity was concerned, then, the doctor seems to have therapeutic activities as a giver of permission, an approver of actions already taken and finally as a person who acts as a reality against which the patient can test self-perceptions and constructs.

There is now a causal model for depression, largely validated by the fundamental work of George Brown and Tirril Harris (1978). They identified in their research, three sets of happenings associated with depressive experience: provoking agents; vulnerability or protective factors; and symptom formation factors. They propose some theoretical interpretation in explanation of their findings.

There is no doubt on considering the model, that it indicates that the activities of the doctor and values of his relationship with the patient, can be utilized to protect patients from depression, or at least to ameliorate the severity of the experience when it occurs.

CONCLUSION

Those trained in the use of the doctor–patient relationship in general practice seem convinced of its value in diagnosis and treatment and believe that proper use of the relationship is one way of increasing the effectiveness of communication between doctor and patient (Balint and Norell, 1973).

If this is accepted then the ways used to train doctors in more effective communication must be studied with care. These can be categorized under two broad headings. The first pertains to a form of reductionism and entails isolating the component skills required for effective communication; the second pertains to a form of holism and entails the acquisition of appropriate perceptions of role, purpose and methods.

The first is a useful precursor for the second. The first can utilize detailed analysis of single performances and a variety of other technical methods (Byrne and Long, 1976). The holistic approach however, is greater than the sum of the items of behaviour which go to make it up. Acquisition of skills in the holistic approach requires these specific behaviours to be deployed with real patients, and preferably going on to discuss in a group of peers the transactions which take place, making predictions, and taking the results back to more work with patients. It is a long, tiring and iterative process. It is part of the continuing education of doctors who will all feel rewarded to know that the relationships they enjoy with their patients can be used altruistically to help patients avoid maladaptive responses and achieve optimum development as individuals.

REFERENCES

Balint, E. and Norell, J. S. (eds) (1973). *Six Minutes for the Patient*. Tavistock Publications, London.
Balint, M. (1957). *The Doctor, His Patient and the Illness*. Pitman Medical, London.
Balint, M., Hunt, J., Joyce, D., Marinker, M. and Woodcock, J. (1970). *Treatment or Diagnosis*. Tavistock Publications, London.
Brown, G. W. and Harris, T. (1978). *Social Origins of Depression*. Tavistock Publications, London.
Browne, K. and Freeling, P. (1976). The Doctor–Patient Relationship. Churchill Livingstone, Edinburgh.
Byrne, P. S. and Long, B. E. (1976). *Doctors Talking to Patients*. Her Majesty's Stationery Office, London.
Festinger, L. (1964). *Conflict, Decision and Dissonance*. Stanford University Press, California.
Freeling, P. (1976). Interactions in small groups. In *Language and Communication in General Practice* (B. A. Tanner, ed.), pp. 180–197. Hodder and Stoughton, London.
Freeling, P. (1978). Those who can. William Pickles Lecture 1978. *J. Roy. Coll. Gen. Pract.* **28**, 329–340.
Freeling, P. (1982). *The Postgraduate Education of General Practitioners in Great Britain* (in press).
Gray, D. J. P. (1977). A System of Training for General Practice, Occasional Paper, No. 4. *J. Roy. Coll. Gen. Pract.*, London.
Greco, R. S. and Pittenger, R. A. (1966). *One Man's Practice*. Tavistock Publications, London.

Hasler, J. C. (1978). Training practices in the Oxford Region. *J. Roy. Coll. Gen. Pract.* 28, 352–354.

Hymes, D. (1972). Models of the interaction of language and social life, in Direction in Sociolinguistics. In *The Ethnography of Communication* (JJ. Gumperz. and D. Hymes, eds). Holt, Rinehart and Winston, New York.

Leeuwenhorst Working Party (1974). The General Practitioner in Europe. The Netherlands: Pamphlet published by the Working Party on the Second European Conference on the Teaching of General Practice. *J. Roy. Coll. Gen. Pract.* 27, 117.

Long, B. (1974). Doctors Talking to Patients: Verbal Communication. *Gen. Pract. Internat.* 4, 152–158.

Marks, J. (1978). *The Benzodiazepines, Use, Overuse, Misuse, Abuse.* pp. 51–57. MTP Press. Lancaster.

Morrell, D. C., Gaze, H. G. and Robinson, N. A. (1970). Patterns of demand in general practice. *J. Roy. Coll. Gen. Pract.* 19, 331–342.

O'Flanagan, P. H. (1977). One trainee's clinical experience. *J. Roy. Coll. Gen. Pract.* 27, 227–230.

Pardes, M. (1977). In *Understanding Human Behaviour in Health and Illness* (R. C. Simons and H. Pardes, eds), pp. 479–484. Williams and Wilkinson, Baltimore.

Royal College of General Practitioners (1972). *The Future General Practitioner—Teaching and Learning.* British Medical Journal, London.

Royal College of General Practitioners (1973). Present state and future needs of general practice (3rd edition). Report from General Practice No. 16. Council of the Royal College of General Practitioners, London.

Royal College of General Practitioners (1977). Better Clinical Standards. Report of a Working Party of the Board of Censors to the Council of the Royal College of General Practitioners, London (privately circulated).

Stimson, G. V. (1978). Interactions between patients and general practitioners in the United Kingdom. In *The Doctor–Patient Relationship in the Changing Health Scene* (E. B. Gallagher, ed.), pp. 69–84. U.S. Department of Health, Education and Welfare.

Szasz, T. and Hollender, M. (1950). A contribution to the philosophy of medicine: the basic models of the doctor–patient relationship. *Arch. Int. Med.* 97, 585.

Tait, I. (1974). Person-centred perspectives in medicine. *J. Roy. Coll. Gen. Pract.* 24, 151–160.

Tallent, N. (1978). *Psychology of Adjustment,* pp. 46–50. Van Norstrand, New York.

Taylor, D. C. (1979). The components of sickness: diseases, illnesses and predicaments. *Lancet* 2, 1008–1010.

Thomson, G. H. (1978). Tolerating uncertainty in family medicine. *J. Roy. Coll. Gen. Pract.* 28, 343–346.

9 Prescribing and the Doctor–Patient Relationship

Ann Cartwright

Kafka's country doctor maintained that: "To write prescriptions is easy, but to come to an understanding with people is hard". This was quoted by Balint *et al.* (1970) in their study of repeat prescriptions in general practice. In this chapter I suggest that the increase in prescribing in recent years is associated with a deterioration in some aspects of the doctor–patient relationship. I present data that suggest a rise in prescribing without consultation and an increase in the proportion of patients not taking the drugs prescribed for them. I argue that many patients have anxieties about taking prescribed drugs which for various reasons they do not communicate to their doctor. Rejecting the doctor's advice covertly but not openly, undermines the doctor–patient relationship.

1 METHODS

In 1969 the Institute for Social Studies in Medical Care did a study of medicine takers, prescribers and hoarders (Dunnell and Cartwright, 1972). A survey with a rather similar design and including a number of comparable questions was carried out in 1977 (Cartwright and Anderson, 1981). Both studies were based on a sample of people on the electoral register in a number of randomly selected parliamentary constituencies. The 1969 study covered England, Wales and Scotland, the 1977 one was confined to England and Wales. The people who were interviewed were asked for the name and address of their doctor and these general practitioners were sent a postal questionnaire. So both studies were concerned with the experiences and views of patients and their doctors. Response rates were rather higher on the more recent study: 84%

of patients responded in 1977 compared with 76% in 1969, and on both studies the response rate of general practitioners was lower: 67% in 1977, 56% in 1969. Another methodological difference was that in 1969 the electoral register was restricted to people aged 21 or over while in 1977 it covered those aged 18 or more.

Questions about prescribed medicines were confined to those which people reported they had taken during the 14 days before the interview, but the way in which the information was elicited on the studies was rather different. In 1969 people were asked about a list of 25 types of medicaments and then for each one they were taking they were asked if they had got it on a doctor's prescription. In 1977 they were asked if they had taken or used any medicines, tablets, ointments or contraceptive pills that were prescribed by a doctor, hospital or clinic.

2 CONSULTATION AND PRESCRIBING RATES

In England and Wales the average number of prescription items dispensed per patient on the N.H.S. rose from 5·60 in 1969 to 6·58 in 1977, an increase of 18% (D.H.S.S. personal communication).

Consultation rates with general practitioners were similar on the 1969 and 1977 studies and data from a number of other studies (discussed in Cartwright and Anderson, 1981) also suggest that there has been little or no change in consultation rates over a number of years. In addition, the proportion of consultations at which a prescription was given was two-thirds on both studies.

How can this evidence be reconciled with national data about the increase in the number of prescription items dispensed? Two possibilities present themselves. One is that doctors have increased the number of items prescribed at a consultation. No information is available from the two surveys to support or refute this. Data from the D.H.S.S. (personal communication) indicate a small rise of 6% in the average number of *items per prescription* from 1·54 in 1969 to 1·63 in 1977. So this may be part of the explanation, but is not enough to account for the 18% rise in prescribing rates.

The second possibility, to account for an increase in the number of prescriptions while consultation rates and the proportion of consultations at which a prescription is issued remain constant, is that the number of prescriptions issued without a direct consultation with the doctor have increased. In 1969 we found that 25% of the prescriptions received in a two week period were obtained without seeing the doctor. In 1977, 39% of the prescribed medicines being taken in a two week period had been obtained without the patient seeing the doctor on the last occasion at which a prescription was obtained. Unfortunately these two figures are not directly comparable. The types of drugs which people take in a two week period are likely to be different from the types prescribed in any two weeks, the former probably including more medicines that had been prescribed over a long period. And the more frequently the same item had been obtained the less likely the patient was to see the doctor. In 1969 14% of repeats which had previously been prescribed four times or less were usually obtained without seeing the doctor. This proportion rose to 41% for items which had been prescribed twenty or more times. In 1977 among prescribed medicines taken in the previous two weeks the proportion for which the last prescription was obtained without seeing a doctor rose from 35% of those for which two–four prescriptions had been given to 67% of those for which 20 or more prescriptions had been received.

The data from our two surveys about changes in the proportion of prescriptions obtained without seeing a doctor are inconclusive but highly suggestive. The increase in receptionists and secretaries during this period (Cartwright and Anderson, 1981) is likely to have made it easier for doctors to issue a prescription without a consultation. And data from two other studies also suggest that the practice may have become more widespread. A study in 1977 by one pharmacist of 2237 prescriptions prescribed by 79 doctors found that 37% of the prescriptions were either wholly or partly written by a receptionist (Jones, 1978). While an earlier study in 1970 of 116 doctors and 86498 prescriptions reported that 10% were written by someone other than the signing doctor (Austin and Parish, 1976).

So the most plausible explanation for the fact that the rise in prescriptions has not been accompanied by an increase in either consultations or the proportion of consultations at which a prescription is given to the patient, is that there has been an increase in the number of prescriptions issued without a direct consultation with the doctor. What are the implications?

3 IMPLICATIONS OF PRESCRIPTIONS WITHOUT CONSULTATION

It has just been shown that those taking medicines on a prescription obtained without seeing the doctor tended to be people on long-term medication. And as would be expected, the more prescribed medicines a person was taking the greater the chance that at least one of the current prescriptions had been obtained without seeing a doctor: the proportion rose from 37% of those taking one medicine to 51% of those taking four or more. In addition prescribed medicine taking increases with age (Dunnell and Cartwright, 1972; Skegg *et al.* 1977; Anderson, 1980b). So among the medicine takers the proportion taking at least one on a prescription obtained without seeing the doctor rose from 18% of those under 25 to 57% of those aged 65 or more. This means that prescriptions without consultations tend to be given more often to those taking multiple drugs and to the elderly. And it is the elderly who are most prone to adverse reactions because of reduced excretion, slower metabolism and also probably increased sensitivity (Williamson, 1978).

The types of medicine most often obtained on prescription without consultation were cardiovascular or diuretic 54%, psychotropic 47% and rheumatic 44%. For the others the proportions varied between 18% and 41% averaging 30%. Again this is to be expected since cardiovascular or diuretic and psychotropic drugs are the ones most likely to be prescribed on a long-term basis (Anderson, 1980a).

Turning to the patients taking medicines, we did not find any difference in their views about their doctors between those who sometimes got their prescription without seeing the doctor and those who saw their doctor every time. They were as likely to regard their doctor as friendly or businesslike, to find him or her easy to talk to and to view their doctor as someone they might consult about a personal matter that was not strictly medical. Neither did the two groups differ in their feelings about whether they knew enough about their medicines. However, it is a matter of some concern that a third of all medicine takers felt that their knowledge of the medicines they took was inadequate.[1] Some comments illustrate that much of the information desired was fairly basic:

I'd like to know what purpose they are for and what they're actually doing for me.

What they do for you—what they're supposed to do for you. You've no idea—you're just taking their recommendation—I'd like to know if there could be side effects.

I'd like to know if I can drink while taking the Equagesic, or what food I should not have.

Altogether, 20% of people taking a prescribed medicine said that the medicine(s) restricted their activities, like drinking or driving, in some way; 5% did not know if there was anything they should or should not do while taking the medicine.[2] And 23% thought there was likely to be some side effects of their drug use, 65% thought not and 12% did not know.[3]

One of the disadvantages of obtaining prescriptions without seeing the doctor is that side effects and drug interactions may not be recognized and these figures suggest that many patients may not be alert to the possibility. Even among those taking oral contraceptives the proportion mentioning the likelihood of side effects, although higher than for other drugs, was still less than half, while the proportion of patients who recognized that there might be any adverse effects from their drug use did not increase with the number of prescribed medicines they were taking.

In another study of consultations between elderly patients and their general practitioners it was found that when patients were taking prescribed medicines in addition to those prescribed at the study consultation, doctors were not aware of this in a third of the instances (Cartwright *et al.*, 1974). It is possible but by no means certain that, when doctors give prescriptions without seeing a patient, their records are kept more carefully. On the other hand it is doubtful if many doctors review the whole prescribing picture for a patient when signing a prescription but not seeing the patient.

To sum up, the evidence suggests that the practice of issuing repeat prescriptions without seeing patients has increased. And it is argued that this is likely to lead to failures of communication about drug interactions and side effects partly because the patients receiving such prescriptions tend to be elderly patients taking more than one drug and partly because doctors are sometimes unaware of the medicines their patients are taking.

4 MEDICINE TAKING AND PRESCRIBING RATES

There is a second disparity between the national figures on prescribing rates and the results from our two studies: while the prescribing rate per person rose by 18% the number of prescribed medicines being taken during a two week period remained unchanged between 1969 and 1977. One possibility is that doctors were prescribing for shorter periods at the later date, but patients' reports of the length of time they had been taking prescribed medicines and the number of prescriptions they had received for the medicines they were taking were very similar (Anderson, 1980b). If there had been an increase in the proportion of prescriptions to be taken on a short-term basis then these distributions should have changed.

Other possible contributory factors are the increase in the proportion of elderly people in the population, a fall in the extent of hospital prescribing, a decrease in the samples from pharmaceutical firms issued by general practitioners and a change in the proportion of medicines consumed by children. Conclusive data on each of these are not available; the effects seem likely to be small.

In my view the most plausible explanation for the disparity is that patients have become increasingly anxious about the dangers of drug-taking and more sceptical about the values, and that more of them are not taking the drugs that doctors prescribe in the quantities in which they are issued. The next section examines the evidence for this assertion and the possible reasons for patients not taking prescribed drugs.

5 CHANGING ATTITUDES TO DRUGS

First there is the evidence that people have become rather more critical of doctors and less willing to accept their advice unquestioningly. In two studies of patients and their general practitioners carried out in 1964 and in 1977 (Cartwright, 1967; Cartwright and Anderson, 1981) we found more patients critical in the later study on eight out of the ten criteria they were asked about. In addition both patients and doctors in 1977 generally thought that patients were more likely to question whether the doctor was right than they were ten years ago. Part of the increase in criticism almost certainly stemmed from higher expectations and standards while an increase in knowledge with a consequent rise in self confidence may well account for the greater willingness to question doctors' decisions and assumptions. We found that nearly three quarters of the general practitioners felt their patients were more knowledge-able about health matters than they had been ten years previously (Cartwright and Anderson, 1981). Another indicator of a change in doctor–patient relationships is that in 1977 a third of the patients thought the prestige of general practitioners had been going down in the last ten years compared with 15% who thought it had gone up.

So by 1977 doctors were on a somewhat lower pedestal and patients were less the passive and uncritical acceptors of their general practitioners' care than they had been in 1964. Between 1964 and 1977 there was a small but significant increase in the proportion of patients who were critical of their doctors for being too inclined to give prescriptions, and in 1977 more patients felt their doctor was guilty of this than felt he or she was too reluctant to give them. The figures are in Table 9.1.

Some comments from those who felt their doctor was too inclined to give a

Table 9.1. Views on doctors' prescribing habits.

	1964	1977
	%	%
Felt doctor was:		
Too inclined to give a prescription	2	7
Rather reluctant to give a prescription	4	4
Reasonable about this	94	89
Number of patients answering questions (=100%)	1159	709

prescription were general:

> You go up there and the first thing he does is write your name on the prescription pad.

> Well you go in, and he never examines you or looks at you, just writes a prescription.

Others were more specific:

> He doesn't even ask you if you want one, he just hands them out. When I had a bad cold, by the time I got to see him it had got a bit better but I needed a certificate for work. He still gave me a full course of penicillin tablets which I didn't think were necessary.

> Three years ago when I had depression after the op. he gave me a prescription for Valium and Tryptizol and I found all I needed was one Tryptizol at night.

Some were more analytical of the doctor's motives:

> I think she gives them just to reassure the patient and not because they are needed.

> I think they always give you a prescription when you go, to make you feel better. They are so busy and have that many patients to see that they haven't really got time to sit down and explain to you that maybe you don't need a prescription if you did this, that or the other, so they just give you one to make you feel better.

When asked about doctors in general many more people expressed criticism about prescription-happy doctors: nearly half, 46%, thought doctors too inclined to give prescriptions, only 2% that they were rather reluctant.

Those who had had a consultation with their doctor in the two weeks before they were interviewed were asked what they had hoped or expected their doctor would do before the consultation.[4] The proportion expecting or hoping for a prescription had declined from 52% in 1964 to 41% in 1977—although the proportion receiving one had not changed. Nearly all those who had hoped for or expected one had been given one, 92%, as had half of those who had not hoped for or expected one.

Evidence that patients do not want prescriptions as often as doctors think they do comes from a variety of sources, some of it anecdotal. Farrant (1980) recorded pregnant women who were prescribed pills but did not take them.

> He (G.P.) gave me some tranquillisers to calm me down, which I've still got. I wouldn't take anything like that when I'm pregnant.

Sheldon, a general practitioner, reported that he started to ask patients for whom a drug might be marginally helpful: "Would you like me to give you something for this?" and was surprised how many said no. In a study of 2182

women who had recently had a baby it was found that four-fifths were offered
or given sleeping tablets during the ten days or so after the birth but a quarter
of these women did not take them (Cartwright, 1979, plus additional
unpublished data).

Stimson (1976) found that general practitioners estimated that a high
proportion of patients expected a prescription: four-fifths of the doctors
believed that prescriptions were expected at 80% or more of consultations and
he contrasts this with studies of patients showing that between a fifth and a half
of them expect a prescription at a consultation.

6 REASONS FOR "EXCESS" PRESCRIBING

Both patient and doctors may be caught up in a circular situation. If general
practitioners respond to what they perceive as patients' wishes for a
prescription, patients may become increasingly likely to *expect* such an
outcome from a consultation. Some support for this comes from an analysis of
how long patients had been with a doctor by whether or not they expected a
prescription. A quarter of patients who had been with the doctor for less than
two years expected a prescription compared with nearly half of those who had
had the same doctor for longer. However, the numbers were small and did not
quite reach the 5% level of significance but the difference could not be attributed
to the age of the patients (Cartwright and Anderson, 1981).

In my view general practitioners are much more likely to realize that a
patient wants a prescription than to recognize that a patient does not want one.
A positive wish is much easier to convey than a negative one. It is relatively
easy to drop hints or to ask outright to be given something for a condition. But
to indicate that a prescription would be unwelcome is difficult to do before it is
given and even more so afterwards: before it seems gratuitous, afterwards it is
rejecting. Patients for the most part want to keep on good terms with their
doctor; to refuse a prescription that is offered, or more generally given without
question, can be seen as insulting.

Another reason why doctors may give a prescription when it is not
necessarily seen as either useful or as wanted, is that the procedure of writing
out the prescription and handing it to the patient is a way of ending a
consultation.

7 IMPLICATIONS OF UNWANTED PRESCRIBING

It can be argued that if patients are given prescriptions which they do not want
then they will not only not take the medicine they will not get the prescription

made up. The evidence suggests that the latter happens relatively rarely. Data from the 1969 study suggested that the proportion was less than 5% (Dunnell and Cartwright, 1972). In Sheldon's practice (1979) the proportion was under 3%. Waters *et al.* (1976) in a study of a mining community found a higher rate of 7%; those least likely to get their prescriptions made up were miners aged 25–34 and it is argued that these men need to consult the doctor in order to get sickness benefit but that the "medical content of the consultation in these circumstances is perceived by them as irrelevant".

Not to get a prescription made up at all is a clear rejection of the doctor's advice. To get it made up but then to take it just once or twice may be seen as a less definite action. At the time of our 1977 study it cost 20p to get each item dispensed but 63% were dispensed free to patients (D.H.S.S., 1978). There is evidence that there are a lot of prescribed medicines lying around in people's homes. In our 1969 study we found that 73% of households had some prescribed medicines and the average number was 3·0. Forty-five per cent of the prescribed medicines had not been used in the month before the interview and 22% had been in people's homes for a year or more. On that study we estimated that around 6% of prescribed medicines were wasted (Dunnell and Cartwright, 1972). It is possible that that proportion was considerably higher in 1977.

So one implication of patients not taking their prescribed drugs or of doctors prescribing in greater quantities than are needed is the waste and cost to the community. Six per cent of the drug bill in Great Britain in 1977 was £40 million (D.H.S.S., 1980). The immediate effect on the patients themselves is questionable. Doubtless there are some for whom it is deleterious and we found on our study of general practitioner consultations with the elderly that doctors were not good at predicting which patients would carry out their advice and which would not (Cartwright, 1976). Presumably if the medicine taking is vital doctors are likely to be aware if it is not being taken. In many situations, however, it may not matter too much that patients are not swallowing all the pills they have been prescribed and for some it could even be an advantage. Law and Chalmers (1976) in their study of medicines and elderly people in one general practice found few patients exceeding the written dose but more patients taking drugs less often than instructed. They reported that "no ill effects were observed from altered regimens".

Is it possible to identify which drugs patients are least likely to take? A comparison of the drugs prescribed in England in 1977 (D.H.S.S., 1980) with the types of drugs adults in our sample were taking in the two weeks before interview shown in Table 9.2 can only provide broad clues about this.

Given the different bases of the two sets of figures the similarity of the two distributions is in many ways surprising. The main differences are over cardiovascular and diuretic drugs, hormone drugs and those acting system-ically on infections. Preparations for treating infections are prescribed

Table 9.2. A comparison of the type of drugs prescribed in England in 1977 with those taken by our sample of adults in 1977.

	Prescriptions dispensed in England in 1977[b] %	Drugs taken by adults in 2 weeks before interview[c] %
Psychotropic drugs[a]	16	17
Other preparations acting on the nervous system	10	10
Preparations acting on the gastrointestinal system	8	5
Preparations acting on the cardio-vascular system and diuretics	14	20
Preparations acting on the respiratory system or affecting allergic reactions	12	9
Preparations prescribed for rheumatism	5	7
Preparations acting systemically on infections	13	6
Preparations with hormone or anti-hormone activity	5	14
Preparations affecting haemopoiesis and the blood and those for nutritional disorders	4	4
Preparations acting on the eye or locally on the skin and mucous membrane	11	8
Other	2	—
Number (=100%)	285 602 000	671[d]

[a] Hypnotics, sedatives and tranquillizers, CNS stimulants and depressant combinations, anti-depressants and anti-depressant and sedative/tranquillizer combinations, appetite suppressants.
[b] Excluding preparations for immunology, preparations used in diagnosis, disinfectants, antiseptics, surgical and industrial spirits, dressings and appliances.
[c] Includes oral contraceptives which is the reason why figures are slightly different from those reported by Anderson, (1980b).
[d] Twenty-nine, 4%, could not be classified and have been excluded.

relatively frequently for children but prescriptions are seldom repeated (Skegg et al., 1977). The disparities over hormonal drugs and over cardiovascular and diuretic drugs are in the opposite direction to that for the infections and could be because prescriptions for these are often repeats given over a long time. These were the drugs most likely to have been prescribed a year or more previously; 79% of people taking cardiovascular or diuretic drugs and 72% of those on hormonal drugs got their first prescription a year or more ago compared with 45% of people taking other types of drugs. But if we consider the proportion of people on different types of drugs the proportions who had been taking them for five years or more were 28% of those on hormonal drugs, 20% of those on cardiovascular and diuretics and 20% of those on psychotropic drugs compared with 13% of those on other drugs. If long-term prescribing accounts for the discrepancies then a similar difference might be expected for psychotropic drugs. Looking at the number of different prescriptions which patients said they had received for the different drugs the proportion who had had ten or more prescriptions was highest for cardiovascular and diuretic drugs, 68%, next for psychotropic, 47%, with hormonal drugs coming third at 46%. And earlier we saw that prescriptions for cardiovascular and diuretic and psychotropic drugs were the ones most likely to be obtained without seeing the doctor.

The pattern of drug prescribing suggests that the proportion of adults taking psychotropic drugs would be higher than the proportion of prescriptions dispensed for these types of drugs—in the same way that there is such a difference for cardiovascular and diuretic drugs and for hormonal ones. A possible explanation for the lack of difference is that patients are less likely to take psychotropic than other sorts of drugs regularly when they are prescribed. The data are certainly no more than suggestive but it seems a plausible hypothesis.

Failure to take some psychotropic drugs when they are prescribed may not always be a bad thing. But a disturbing victim of "excess" prescribing is the quality of the doctor–patient relationship. The rest of this chapter is devoted to justifying this statement.

8 "EXCESS" PRESCRIBING AND THE DOCTOR–PATIENT RELATIONSHIP

For patients to reject the doctor's advice and help by not taking all the medicine that he or she has prescribed, indicates some alienation. This may stem from the doctor's assumption that a patient wants a prescription, without finding out whether this is so or not. Most patients want to be involved in the decision-making process. When a random sample of over 2000 women who had recently had a baby were asked: "If there is any doubt about which of two things a doctor should do for you would you prefer him to decide without telling you or would you rather he explained and let you choose?", the great majority, 81%, said they would rather he explained and let them choose, and three-quarters or more of women in all social classes held this view (Cartwright, 1979).

It is possible that when patients are not involved in the decision to prescribe a drug they are less likely to take it—the lack of involvement makes the rejection of the doctor's advice more likely. The process of alienation starts with the lack of involvement in the decision but is likely to go beyond the rejection of the medicine. If the patient does not take the drug the alienation will be reinforced by the outcome—whatever it is. If the patient gets better as quickly or more quickly than expected this confirms that the medicine was unnecessary. If the patient gets worse, or takes longer than expected to recover, this will be because the doctor gave the wrong treatment or failed to convince the patient that the treatment advised was appropriate. It is the opposite situation to that of the proverbial doctor who always expresses grave doubts about a patient's condition; whatever the outcome it reflects advantageously on the doctor's skill: his diagnostic skill if the patient dies, his therapeutic skill should the patient recover.

The act of rejection itself undermines the doctor–patient relationship from the patient's point of view. Patients tend to accept and make the best of the help and advice their doctors give them. They want to feel they can trust their doctor's judgement, and to respect his or her professionalism. To go to the length of rejecting the specific advice he or she has given to them undermines that sense of trust and the security it engenders. It will not be done lightly but once it has been done may have far-reaching repercussions.

It can be argued that when a patient rejects a doctor's advice, the relationship is more equal than when the patient accepts the advice without questioning it. But by simply not taking the medicine the patient is not rejecting the advice openly. Accepting the prescription but not taking the medicine can be seen as the worst of both worlds. The patient does not feel equal enough to question the doctor directly; the doctor's authority or professionalism is not openly challenged. Appearances are preserved but the doctor cannot learn from the experience. The relationship has deteriorated into a ritual which is in danger of becoming more and more meaningless. The earlier tendency for patients to trust their doctors without question has not yet been replaced with a more satisfying relationship in which doubts can be raised, assumptions challenged and questions answered.

Patients who thought their doctor was too inclined to give prescriptions may have felt they were given a prescription rather than an examination or information or discussion. This is suggested by the analyses in Table 9.3 (Cartwright and Anderson, 1981).

There is evidence from the doctor's point of view as well that prescribing, particularly multiple prescribing, is an unsatisfactory substitute for an appropriate doctor–patient relationship. In the study of general practitioner consultations with the elderly we found that fewer medicines were prescribed when the doctor found the patient easy to talk to and that the doctor prescribed fewer medicines when he or she regarded the consultation as very satisfactory (Cartwright, 1974).

Table 9.3. Patients' views of doctors who are too inclined to give prescriptions and those who were reasonable or reluctant about this.

	Patient regards own doctor as:	
	Too inclined to give prescription	Reluctant or reasonable about giving prescription
Would have liked more information about last problem for which consulted doctor	34%	19%
Some occasion in last twelve months when felt doctor might have done more thorough exam[a]	33%	10%
Would like 10 minutes uninterrupted conversation with a sympathetic doctor	38%	21%
Number of patients (=100%)	36	547

[a] Those who had not consulted in the last twelve months have been excluded.

Patients who take many prescribed medicines may develop a dependency on their doctor. In the 1969 study people were asked if they would consult their doctor in six hypothetical situations. The proportion who were taking prescribed medicine rose from 20% of those who said they would not consult a doctor in any of the six situations to 62% of those who would seek the doctor's advice about all of them (Dunnell and Cartwright, 1972). It may simply be that people who are relatively likely to regard it as appropriate to consult a doctor consult more in practice and this results in more medicines being prescribed for them. But taking drugs can be habit forming (quite apart from addictive) and may therefore lead to more frequent consultation and so engender feelings of dependency.

The only apparent beneficiary from the situation is the pharmaceutical industry. But the benefits for it may be of short duration. Iatrogenic disease and the dangers of drug interactions are attracting more and more publicity. Heightened awareness of these hazards may lead to a backlash in which many people will be reluctant to take any drugs including those which could help them.

9 IN CONCLUSION

Although I have quoted many findings in support of my arguments much of the interpretation is speculative and subjective. What is certain is that the financial cost of the drugs that general practitioners prescribe is greater than the financial cost of the explanations, listening, advice, home visits and support that they give their patients. My basic contention is that many patients would like to be more involved in the decision-making process that takes place at a consultation; they would like, and they often need, more information— and fewer drugs.

ACKNOWLEDGEMENTS

I am indebted to past and present colleagues particularly to Robert Anderson, Karen Dunnell, Sue Lucas, Maureen O'Brien and Christopher Smith. I am also grateful to members of the Institute's Advisory Committee for their help and support over the years, to the many patients and professionals who answered our questions and made the studies possible, to Maureen Roberts and her colleagues at the Department of Health and Social Security, to Jasper Woodcock who commented at various stages, to Danny Kushlick who checked the figures and statements, to Irene Browne who typed this report and to the Department of Health and Social Security who funded most of the Institute for Social Studies in Medical Care studies quoted.

NOTES

1. "Do you feel you know enough about the medicines—what they are and how they are likely to help? IF NO what would you like to know?"
2. "Is there anything you should or should not do while taking this/these medicine(s)?"
3. "Are they likely to have any side effects?"
4. "Before you consulted the G.P. that time what did you think or hope he might do for you? Anything else?"

REFERENCES

Anderson, R. (1980a). The use of repeatedly prescribed medicines. *J. Roy. Coll. Gen. Pract.* **30**, 609–613.
Anderson, R. (1980b). Prescribed medicines: who takes what? *J. Epidemiol. Commun. Hlth.* **34**, 299–304.
Austin, R. and Parish, P. (1976). Prescriptions written by ancillary staff. In *Prescribing in General Practice. J. Roy. Coll. Gen. Pract.* Supplement No. 1, **26**, 24–31.
Balint, M., Hunt J., Joyce, D., Marinker, M. and Woodcock, J. (1970). *Treatment or*

Diagnosis: A Study of Repeat Prescriptions in General Practice. Tavistock Publications, London.

Cartwright, A. (1967). *Patients and their Doctors.* Routledge and Kegan Paul, London.

Cartwright, A. (1974). Prescribing and the relationship between patients and doctors. In *Social Aspects of the use of Psychotropic Drugs* (R. Cooperstock, ed.). Addiction Research Foundation of Ontario, Toronto.

Cartwright A. (1976). What goes on in the general practitioner's surgery?. In *Seminars in Community Medicine, Volume 1 Sociology* (R. M. Acheson and L. Aired, eds). Oxford University Press, Oxford.

Cartwright, A. (1979). *The Dignity of Labour?* Tavistock Publications, London.

Cartwright, A. and Anderson, R. (1981). *General Practice Revisited.* Tavistock Publications, London.

Cartwright, A., Lucas, S. and O'Brien, M. (1974). Exploring Communication in General Practice. A Pilot Study. Cyclostyled.

Department of Health and Social Security. (1978). *Annual Report for 1977.* H.M.S.O., London.

Department of Health and Social Security. (1980). *Health and Personal Social Services Statistics for England 1978.* H.M.S.O., London.

Dunnell, K. and Cartwright, A. (1972). *Medicine Takers, Prescribers and Hoarders.* Routledge and Kegan Paul, London.

Farrant, W. (1980). Importance of Counselling in Antenatal Screening. *Mims,* June 55–63, London.

Jones, D. R. (1978). Errors on doctors' prescriptions. *J. Roy. Coll. Gen. Pract.* **28**, 543–545.

Law, R. and Chalmers, C. (1976). Medicines and elderly people: a general practice survey. *Brit. Med. J.* **1**, 565–568.

Sheldon, M. G. (1979). Self-audit of prescribing habits and clinical care in general practice. *J. Roy. Coll. Gen. Pract.* **29**, 703–711.

Skegg, D. G. G., Doll, R. and Perry, J. (1977). Use of medicines in general practice. *Brit. Med. J.* **1**, 1561.

Stimson, G. V. (1976). Doctor–patient interaction and some problems for prescribing. In *Prescribing in general practice. J. Roy. Coll. Gen. Pract.* Supplement No. 1. **26**, 88–96.

Waters, W. H. R., Gould, N. V. and Lunn, J. E. (1976). Undispensed prescriptions in a mining general practice. *Brit. Med. J.* **1**, 1062–1063.

Williamson, J. (1978). Prescribing problems in the elderly. *Practitioner* **220**, 749–755.

10   *Communicating with Elderly People*

Muir Gray

1 BELIEFS AND ATTITUDES

Communication with older people presents problems for many professionals not just because the prevalence of auditory, visual and speech impairment is higher in older age groups but also because the beliefs and attitudes of older people are different from those of younger people. Their beliefs and attitudes always have to be taken into account, particularly in interviews which result from referral by a third party who has identified a problem which the old person refuses to recognize.

1.1 Beliefs

1.1.1 *Ageism*

Some old people say "I'm all right" and refuse offers of help because they believe that their physical deterioration is an inevitable consequence of the ageing process—"what else can you expect at my age?"—which they know to be untreatable. Regrettably, this belief has often been reinforced by doctors who have asked questions such as "What else do you expect? You are eighty-four after all". It is true that some of the problems which affect older people cannot be cured but this should only be accepted after a thorough medical examination has excluded the possibility that an elderly person's physical, psychological or social problems result from a treatable disease.

Because they attribute all symptoms to ageing, many elderly people do not seek help until their condition has become very severe. Furthermore, even when an older person has referred himself or has been referred by a third party and has a treatable cause for his problem diagnosed, he may not believe the doctor who tells him that his problems can be cured or alleviated and fail to comply with his advice. Ageist beliefs have an important influence on compliance.

1.1.2 *Religious fatalism*

Some old people believe that God caused them to become ill; others that He let it happen, although He did not cause it directly. Some identify a reason why God has allowed this to happen, for example some sin committed many years before, but others cannot identify any reason why they should suffer and are puzzled and either distressed by or resigned to His Will. This type of belief is particularly important not only because it can influence the person's willingness to seek help and to follow advice. Religious beliefs can also affect the efficacy of treatment because distress caused by the belief that his problem is in some way a retribution for past sins can cause depression and make his suffering more severe. For example, analgesics may be less effective because the old person is agitated and distressed by the belief that the reason why he is in pain must be that it is God's Will (Gray 1981).

1.2 Attitudes

1.2.1 *Pessimism*

As a group, very elderly people are more pessimistic because their generation has experienced so many disappointments. They went willingly to fight the "War to End All Wars", having been promised that it would be "over by Christmas" and that there would be "Homes Fit for Heroes", none of which proved true. More disappointment followed in the twenties and thirties—culminating in the promise of "Peace in Our Time" which was followed by another war. If a person becomes disabled he may become more pessimistic, not only because he is promised services which do not materialize, but also because progressive disability is marked by a series of failures. The person is first unable to walk to the shops, then becomes unable to reach the front gate and may eventually fail to reach the front door.

Because of this it may be very difficult to convince the old person that something can be done about his problem, even though he is prepared to accept that it is the result of a treatable disease and not an inevitable consequence of ageing (Gray and Wilcock, 1981).

1.2.2 Fatalism

For some elderly people the best means of preventing the feelings of depression and disillusionment which follow disappointment is to "look on the bright side", reminding oneself that "there are others who are worse off than me" and to keep telling oneself and other people that "I'm all right". This is a more optimistic outlook but it may also cause difficulties with communication because the old person may not want to discuss her problems or consider taking steps to alleviate them. The old person may become fatalistic as a means of coping with the anxiety which his vulnerable and precarious position in the community generates. An elder who is anxious about whether or not he will fall, or become incontinent, or run up debts, or have to go to live in a home, may refuse to discuss these possibilities and the means by which they could be prevented. Instead he reiterates that "there's a bullet with your number on it", or some similar phrase, and this type of fatalistic attitude is not derived from a religious belief but is a means of coping with anxiety, which anthropologists would term magical.

1.2.3 Fear

The declaration "I'm all right" may also be used with the objective of deceiving other people because the old person is afraid. Doctors, like many other professionals, believe that their approach, the information gathered and its interpretation is "objective", whereas relatives, neighbours and the old person give "subjective" information and interpretation. However, only part of the information collected by a professional is verifiable if a strict epistemological definition of the term is used. Certain bits of information gathered by the professional are subjective; that is they are expressions of the person's feeling which cannot be falsified, such as an old person's statement that he needs to go to the toilet or that he is not in pain. Other bits of information are objective, that is their truth can be falsified; for example an old person's statement that he has an inside toilet can be tested by going to see whether or not he has an inside toilet. There is, however, a third type of information which is neither subjective nor objective and it has been called interpersonal information. For example the statement of an old person who lives alone that he can manage to reach the toilet without help is a piece of interpersonal information. It is neither a subjective expression of the old person's feelings or sensations like her statement that she needs to go to the toilet; nor is it an objective, falsifiable, statement like his statement that he has an inside toilet. The old person can be asked if he will show the doctor how he gets to the toilet but he can confound this test by saying that he "doesn't feel up to it just now". Even if evidence that he cannot manage to reach the toilet without help is given by his family, he is able to confound it by saying that he "doesn't like to go to the toilet" when they are there and that he often goes when he is alone.

It is uncommon for old people to lie but they may be very selective about which bits of information they will release and impart a bias to that which is released. Interpersonal information is biased by the person who releases it to achieve a certain objective; for example to impress, mislead or confuse the recipient. In the case of an old person the objective is often to stay at home and "I'm all right" may be stated as a means of achieving that objective or the old person may adopt other strategies.

Miss B. was 82, fiercely independent and prepared to fight for her right to stay on in her sheltered flat. She was eventually admitted to hospital, to the relief of everyone, but recovered and was discharged, as she wished, after much opposition and to the distress of everyone. She was visited at home by the medical social worker, the nursing officer, a representative of the housing association and a doctor. The intention was to "make her see the reality of the situation" which each failed to do individually.

> Social worker (confidently): "Hello Miss B., we've come to see how you're getting on. How are you managing?"
> Miss B. (calmly looking out of the window): "No comment."
> Social worker (less confidently): "Can you get to the toilet?"
> Miss B.: "No comment."
> Social worker (very uncertain how to proceed): "Um, can you make a cup of tea?"
> Miss B. (still calmly looking out of the window): "No comment."
> The professionals retreated in disarray and regrouped outside the flat where the nursing officer said: "She's very confused isn't she?"

Fear of isolation also influences communication and an old person whose home help and district nurse have become friends as well as being professional helpers may bias his information. He may try to conceal the fact that he is improving, exaggerate his difficulties and fail to comply with treatment because he is afraid that the home help and district nurse will be stopped if he becomes independent in the kitchen and bathroom.

2 ETHICAL AND PRACTICAL IMPLICATIONS

These beliefs and attitudes have to be considered and explored but this presents ethical problems. Should the doctor try to persuade the old person to become dissatisfied with his lot and to agree to struggle to achieve some improvement or, to be more accurate, the possibility of some improvement, with the possibility of disappointment and depression if he should fail to achieve the goal which is set, or should he respect the elderly person's beliefs and let him be? The obese old person suffering from disabilities which partly result from his obesity but who maintains that it is impossible to lose weight "at my age" offers one example of this type of dilemma. How far should a doctor go in trying to make him appreciate that the cause of his obesity is within his control? The acceptance of this relationship is necessary before the patient will comply with advice but it may make him feel inadequate if he is unable to lose weight, guilty when he eats energy rich food, and spoil one of his few remaining pleasures.

The ethical dilemma is even more difficult if the person is seriously ill and refuses investigation or treatment.

Mr A. was 74. After the death of the sister with whom he lived he moved into a room in a multi-occupied house. He collapsed in the street and was taken to hospital where he had an operation to stop the bleeding from a gastric ulcer. Two days after discharge he fell at home and twisted his knee. Because he was unable to walk he lay on his bed.

At the time of this referral he had been in bed for three weeks and the mattress was soaked in urine and covered in excrement. A schizophrenic lodger in the next room had boiled eggs for him but as his wallet had been stolen by someone who had come into his room he had not eaten for some days. Even after he had been bathed and given a new mattress it was evident that he required treatment in hospital but he refused to go. He was neither depressed nor demented; he said he did not want to die and wanted to walk again but refused to go to hospital saying "things could be worse" and that there was nothing which could be done. Eventually he was compulsorily removed to hospital using Section 47 of the 1948 National Assistance Act which allows the removal of people suffering from grave chronic disease or who are living in "insanitary conditions" if they are not receiving proper care and attention (Gray 1980). He recovered in hospital and is now enjoying life in the Church Army Hostel.

The precise nature of one's approach should be determined by the beliefs and attitudes of the particular individual who is being interviewed but there are a number of simple guidelines which should be emphasized in professional training.

(1) At an early stage in the interview explain the difference between ageing and disease processes.

(2) Reiterate this difference when specific problems resulting from disease are being discussed and when prescribing medication or giving advice intended to alleviate the problem.

(3) Emphasize the distinction between ageing and disease when treatment or progress is being reviewed.

(4) Remember the religious dimension and help the old person re-establish links with the Church if these have been broken.

(5) Discuss the possibility of failure with the old person and emphasize that

because his problems have increased in recent years this does not mean that his social problems are inevitably unsolvable or will inevitably deteriorate.

(6) Be positive and encouraging, emphasize that she will be able to cope better with her disabilities.

(7) Set specific goals which the old person should be able to attain and reinforce an optimistic attitude by emphasizing the importance of any goal which is achieved as evidence that the person can succeed in spite of his age.

(8) Assume a fear of permanent institutionalization and assure the old person explicitly that "I'm interested in helping you live on in your own home, that's the best place for you" early on in the interview.

3 THIRD PARTY REFERRALS

Often it is necessary to communicate with people other than the old person and their beliefs about old people and public services and their attitudes towards them also have to be taken into account, particularly in cases in which other people are convinced that the old person has a problem but the old person himself maintains that he is "all right".

3.1 Beliefs

Many people hold ageist beliefs. They believe that all very elderly people are of declining intelligence: some even believe that all old people are "dementing". The consequence of such beliefs is that they assume that the old person whom they have referred is unable to appreciate the severity of his problems and expect the professional to whom they have referred the case to "make him see the reality of the situation", that is to say their view of the reality of the situation. People who hold ageist beliefs may also be reluctant to accept that the old person should not be permanently admitted to an institution because they do not believe that any old people can improve, learn new ways of coping or be rehabilitated. Furthermore, the person who has referred the case to the professional may have assumed that the professional will share his view that the old person "needs looking after" and that the best means of doing this will be permanent institutionalization. Many people, however, are not aware of the full range of services which are available and do not understand the contribution which services such as physiotherapy or occupational therapy can make (Gray and Wilcock, 1981a).

3.2 Attitudes

One of the most difficult attitudes is not indifference but over-protection. Not infrequently the professional's principal problem is the anxiety of people other than the older person. Anxiety is often understandable and can be the reason why other people wish to help but it can become counter-productive. When it becomes too great for relatives, neighbours or friends to bear they may take steps such as trying to interfere with people who are providing domiciliary services—"if you stop helping her to live at home, they have to do something"—and phoning the press as well as applying great pressure to the old person himself to agree to go into a home. The result of this can be that the old person becomes paranoid.

The reason for the over-protective attitude is often guilt. People know that they could do more themselves to help the old person but are not willing to make the necessary sacrifices to do so, partly because the needs of the old person are of lower priority than other demands on their time but also because of their attitude towards the public services.

Some people, particularly those who are in insecure jobs, are hostile towards public servants whom they see in secure, well paid, superannuated jobs with "perks" such as travelling allowances and good holidays. Such people often hold the opinion that it is the job of the public services to care for elderly people—"What are we paying all these rates and taxes for?"—and become angry when the professional to whom they have referred the case appears unwilling to help, not only by refusing to institutionalize the old person but also by appearing to expect them to do more for the old person themselves.

3.3 Practical implications

Professionals in training can be given a number of guidelines to help them analyse third party referrals. At the time the referral is made they should try to establish the following points:

(1) Who is anxious about the old person and what are their specific anxieties?

(2) What factors have influenced the timing of the referral—has it been a deterioration in the condition of the elder or a change in the circumstances or condition of someone else?

(3) What does the old person know about the referral?

(4) What does the referrer expect to happen as a result of referral?

When interviewing people who are concerned about the old person the professional should try to learn about their beliefs and attitudes. In professional training it should be emphasized that the following steps are important.

(1) Emphasize the distinction between disease and ageing to the supporters of the old person as well as to the old person himself, emphasizing in particular

that ageing and dementia are distinct processes. If the old person develops dementia point out that it is even more important to prevent isolation and sensory deprivation than before and that people with dementia may become depressed, and anxious and emotional needs are often overlooked when dementia has been diagnosed.

(2) Establish the expectations of other people about the contribution of public services and their own role by discussing their beliefs about, and attitudes towards, public services.

(3) Try to assess how much feelings of guilt contribute towards the attitudes of relatives, friends and neighbours.

4 PROFESSIONAL BELIEFS AND ATTITUDES

Many professionals are as ageist and over-protective at the end of their professional training as they were at the beginning. Medical training, in particular, makes little attempt to modify the attitudes of students towards elderly people, but other professional curricula are little better and ageism and over-protection often influence professional practice. A doctor with ageist attitudes may not examine an old person thoroughly because he ascribes her symptoms to "her age" and a community nurse who is over-protective may put undue pressure on an old person to enter her home as a means of alleviating her own anxiety but professionals are, in general, less prejudiced than untrained people. However, professionals have esoteric beliefs and attitudes which influence their communication with elderly people.

4.1 Hostility

Social surveys have found that old people are more satisfied with their health, housing and other aspects of life than younger people even though their material and physical conditions are worse. Elderly people have lower expectations, make fewer demands, are more easily satisfied and are more grateful largely because of the experience of their generation (Age Concern, 1977). Because they are, in general, more grateful and less demanding it might be thought that they would be a popular group with professionals but this is not the case. They are an unpopular group and this is reflected in a number of ways, notably in the names which are used to describe them in the hospital service—for example "rubbish", "crumble" and "grot".

The reasons for this attitude are first that it may be impossible to diagnose or assess the old person's problem precisely. Secondly, the old person's problem may be, or may wrongly be assumed to be, intractable; and thirdly even if intervention is attempted the results are often slow to become apparent or very difficult to perceive. Most professionals find clients whose problems they can understand and tackle effectively, or whose problems they think they can understand and tackle effectively, much more rewarding than those whose problems they find incomprehensible and intractable.

Two other factors may make professionals hostile towards elderly clients. First the higher prevalence of visual, speech and hearing impairment means that communication between professional and client is more often impeded than when working with younger people. The frustration which may result from this may lead to a loss of interest in the person's problems or even an angry dismissal of the old person as being "too knocked off" or "impossible to talk to". This occurs particularly with elderly people with impairment of hearing or speech.

Secondly, the fact that a higher proportion of clients are seen as a result of third party referrals, as opposed to self-referral, means that a higher proportion of elderly people are suspicious of professionals, particularly of those whom they had never encountered before the visit which follows the referral by the third party. The justifiable suspicions of the old person may lead him to be labelled as "difficult", "aggressive" or even "paranoid".

4.2 Suspicion of relatives

Many professionals believe that the modern family does not care for its elders as well as families did in the past. They believe, as is generally believed, that all old people were loved, respected, and cared for in the past. This was not the case as social historians, notably Keith Thomas (1976), Peter Laslett (1968) and M. J. Moroney (1976) and David Fischer (1977) have clearly demonstrated. However, the belief that the typical modern family is uncaring gives rise to hostile and occasionally punitive attitudes.

The professional who believes this will be on the defensive when communicating with relatives because he suspects that the family are conspiring to get the older person into hospital, and this may influence his communication with them. He may, for example, suspect that their distress is simulated or that their statement that they are exhausted is untrue and he may take their anger and hostility, which actually results from his manner towards them, as evidence that they are uncaring rather than perceiving them to be the consequences of their frustration at his own insensitivity. Furthermore, a professional who believes that all relatives are potential "granny-dumpers" may be reluctant to arrange day care or an admission of limited duration to a hospital or home because he is afraid that "they won't have him back". Some families do reject their elderly relatives but often because they have been offered too little help too late, and the reason this occurs is only partly due to an absolute shortage of resources. It is often due to the attitude of professionals who control the allocation of resources (Isaacs, 1971).

4.3 Implications for Professional Education

In the previous sections of this chapter the importance of ensuring that professionals in training were given adequate teaching on the beliefs and attitudes of elderly people and their supporters was emphasized. However, it is more difficult to put the implications of this section on professional beliefs and attitudes into practice. The beliefs and attitudes of other people are not threatening subjects and groups of trainees can discuss them easily and freely. However, the exposure of the trainee's own mistaken beliefs or prejudices about elderly people and their families is a much more difficult topic which may be very threatening to the professional. It may therefore require the trainee to be given time alone with his tutor and the tutor will require careful preparation before discussing these topics because the content of such a tutorial may involve personal counselling as well as an intellectual analysis of beliefs and attitudes and the manner in which they may influence the professional's practice.

This whole subject is discussed elsewhere in the book but a list of the type of topics which should be covered in tutorials which have the objective of preparing the trainee for communicating with elderly people is included in this chapter.

(1) Does the trainee have ageist attitudes?

(2) Does he feel over-protective towards elderly people? If so is it because of an ageist belief that elderly people often don't know what's best for them, or is it because he finds cases in which old people are at risk make him very anxious? A useful focus for discussion is his attitude towards suicide and euthanasia.

(3) How much is he influenced by the attitude of an elderly person and her supporters towards him?

A professional can be trained to make allowances for the mistaken beliefs and biased attitudes of other people but he has to be educated in the fullest sense of the word if he is to be able to appreciate and make allowances for his own mistaken beliefs and prejudices.

REFERENCES

Age Concern (1977). *Profiles of the Elderly: Aspects of Life Satisfaction.* Vol. 1, pp. 31–48. Age Concern, London.

Fischer, D. H. (1977). *Growing Old in America.* Oxford.

Gray, J. A. M. (1980). Section 47: An Ethical Dilemma for Doctors. *Health Trends* **12**, 72–74.

Gray, J. A. M. (1981). Caring for Religious Aspects of Disability. *The Times*, Saturday, February 7th.

Gray, J. A. M. and Wilcock, G. K. (1981a). *Our Elders*, pp. 48–60. Oxford.

Gray, J. A. M. and Wilcock, G. K. (1981b). *Our Elders*, pp. 26–47. Oxford.

Isaacs, B. (1971). Geriatric Patients—do their families care? *Brit. Med. J.* **4**, 282–286.

Laslett, P. (1968). *The World We Have Lost.* Methuen, London

Moroney, M. H.(1976). *The Family and the State.* Longmans, Harlow.

Thomas, K. V. (1976). *Age and Authority in Early Modern England.* Proceedings of the British Academy, Vol. 62.

11   Patient Participation

Peter Pritchard

1 INTRODUCTION

Much of this book is concerned with face-to-face contact between patients and general practitioners in the consulting room. This is natural, because the general practitioner spends about half his time in this way. But communication has many facets, and in this chapter I hope to describe a number of different ways in which patients and general practitioners communicate. The main emphasis will be on Patient Participation which has been developing in England and Wales since 1972 (Paine 1974; Pritchard, 1975, 1979; Wilson, 1975).

But first we must be clear about what we mean by a patient, and whether there is a "patient's point of view" to which doctors can listen for their own advantage as well as their patients' (see Section 2).

The general practitioner is part of a very complicated system for providing primary health care. Other professional health workers (such as community nurses and health visitors) are involved, and their contributions are essential. However, most people will agree that the general practitioner holds (or should hold) the key to successful care. He is responsible for diagnosis, for referral of the majority of patients to hospital, and nearly all prescribing. He is the focal point for a large number of messages to and from a wide range of agencies. He is part of a number of local networks which may or may not involve his patients. Likewise his patients spend most of their time in networks which are not specifically to do with health care. Yet preoccupation with health is very widespread. Thus any attempt to describe and classify patient–general practitioner communication is very difficult. An attempt to do this in terms of "level" (from individual to national) and "pathways" is made in Section 3. It is of necessity incomplete, and excludes the actual consultation which is the topic of other chapters.

In Sections 4 and 5 the development of patient participation is described. The present position is outlined, its varieties and functions are described. An attempt is made to assess its value in negotiating the limits and meeting the aims of primary health care, and in helping health care to adapt to change.

If patient participation is considered to be a useful part of primary health care, then thought must be given to the implications for medical and paramedical training and research (see Section 6).

2 THE PATIENT'S VIEW OF PRIMARY HEALTH CARE

Before discussing the patient's view of the care he receives, we need to be clear about what we mean by a "patient". The dictionary definition of "one who suffers" or "is having medical care" does not cover all current usage. Two distinct meanings have emerged, one implying that the subject is ill and is accepting a sick role and the other that the individual is on the list of a doctor who accepts responsibility for his medical care should he become ill, or be at risk of becoming ill.

These definitions apply to two very different populations in the setting of general practice in the United Kingdom. A patient (sick person) has definite feelings about the health care he (or she) is receiving. He may have suggestions, or grumbles or complaints; or, as is more likely, he is moderately or very satisfied with the service he is receiving. It would be easier to motivate him to join a "patient group", while he was ill, than when he was better.

The patient (person on doctor's list) who does not happen to be ill, may not see himself as a patient at all and may not be keen to join a patient group unless driven by past experience, or concern about friends or relatives, or seeing it as his duty as a citizen not as a patient. The former group might be more concerned with the quality of care being experienced: the latter with access to health care. Good access and good quality do not necessarily go hand in hand, as pointed out in "Access to Primary Care" (H.M.S.O., 1979).

In the United Kingdom, where everyone has the opportunity to register with a general practitioner and 98% do so, the second use of the word patient is becoming more common. It is the meaning used in particular by general practitioners. For those doctors who see their role applying to all their patients, not just those who knock on their door, the distinction becomes less important.

The implications of the National Health Service (N.H.S.) list of patients are far reaching. It gives the general practitioner a list of people for whose medical care he is responsible. It also gives him an opportunity to prevent illness, and to educate his patients to use existing services effectively. This change of emphasis towards prevention implies a shift in the general practitioner's role from the "doctor" as counsellor and therapist towards the doctor as a provider and *manager* of services. The doctor in his manager role will need different information from his patients and different ways of communicating with them.

In rural areas the boundaries of the community and the practice are likely to be much the same. In large towns the doctor may not be part of his local community, nor be so aware of factors affecting the health of the population for which he is responsible. This may be a serious barrier to communication, particularly in deprived inner cities with a high patient turnover.

Should this matter? Does the general practitioner need to know what his patients are thinking and feeling—not just about medical care, but about life and death, about work and leisure, about happiness and despair? Some general practitioners argue that they learn enough about this from their daily contacts with individual patients, and there is no doubt that a general practitioner who listens to his patients has an unrivalled store of social information. But does this sum of knowledge gained from individuals when they are ill give a clear picture of the life and stresses in the community? It can only apply to those who come for medical care (see Hannay, 1979), and the communication is coloured by the anxieties generated by the illness, the consultation and the pressure of time. Patients when ill are reluctant to talk about difficulties of access or acceptability: they do not want to upset the doctor, nor divert him from their objective for the consultation. Outside the consultation, patients raise different topics and give different answers. It is no surprise that a wide range of topics is discussed in Patient Participation Groups (Pritchard, 1978) which are unlikely to be mentioned in a busy consulting session.

Anyone who listens in a public house or bus queue (or watches television) will be aware of the community's intense preoccupation with health topics. Strong opinions are held about every detail. Should general practitioners and their staff be aware of these feelings of their patients? Do they need some feedback? Can they learn something useful from their patients? Can they use this great source of interest and energy to improve health and health care? If the answer is yes to any of these questions, we must consider how we can obtain this information, and tap this source of energy. This will be considered in Sections 4 and 5, but first it might be useful to consider briefly some of the pathways of communication between patients and doctors and the levels at which these operate. This is the topic of the next section, which is summarized in Table 11.1.

3 LEVELS AND PATHWAYS OF COMMUNICATION

Information passes between patients and doctors by many different pathways

Table 11.1 Levels and pathways of patient–doctor communication.

Level	Pathways
Individual (one-to-one)	pre-access access and reception consultation surveillance and recall
small group	pre-access home visits self-help groups
Neighbourhood	informal contacts community services and networks
Practice	handouts/notices/lectures therapeutic groups Patient Participation Group (PPG)
Institutional and district	Family Practitioner Committee (complaints) Community Health Council consumer groups/local radio phone-ins
National (many with local branches)	disease/disability organizations consumer organizations community organizations media research studies of patients' attitudes

at many different levels. It would be difficult to list them all, but an attempt is made in Table 11.1 to include those of major relevance to the general practitioner. Of those the following will be discussed in this or later sections: (a) Pre-access; (b) Access and reception; (c) Doctor-initiated communication; (d) Patient participation groups PPGs (See Sections IV and V); (e) Community Health Councils; (f) Organizations at national level.

3.1 Pre-access

Several writers have described the activity and heart-searching which goes on before an individual seeks help from a general practitioner (Suchman, 1966; Robinson, 1971; Wright, 1978). Though this is not strictly patient–doctor communication it affects the decision to consult or not to consult. Doctors should know about it and it should be accessible to educational influence. The need for this is starkly revealed in a recent study of people who should be seeing a doctor, but fail to do so—the "symptom iceberg" (Hannay, 1979, 1980).

There are many elements in the decision to consult: the presence of a symptom; its significance to the individual with consequent anxiety; the influence of family, friends and lay advisers upon whether and where to seek help; the level of anxiety in the community; the accessibility and likely acceptability of professional help; and the individual's reluctance to bother the doctor, or to accept a sick role. The general practitioner may feel powerless to influence this process from his surgery chair—apart from ensuring that he provides an accessible and acceptable service. If, however, he lives in the community he serves, he will be sensitive to the nuances of anxiety caused by events outside the field of health care. Certain groups, such as adolescents and the elderly, are notoriously reluctant to consult, and informal contacts may help to break down the barrier. This is more difficult in a city setting where the doctor may not live in the practice area.

As a long-term measure, a practice can educate its patients in what to expect—when to see a doctor and when to treat themselves. This takes time and effort which becomes excessive where the patient turnover is high.

The primary care service is the portal of entry (in the United Kingdom) for nearly all hospital care, and so is (or should be) of concern to the hospital service. There is a parallel between the general practitioner and his "pre-access" patients and between the hospital and its referral process. Appropriate referral should be a key issue for hospitals, yet we know that referral rates by individual general practitioners vary enormously (R.C.G.P., 1978) (Last, 1967). This variation has been little studied nor understood in spite of its importance as the "raw material input" to hospitals. Does a similar discrepancy exist in the population of patients who consult a general practitioner? Apart from Hannay's careful study we have little quantitative data about what goes on beyond the normally accepted entrance to primary health care—the reception desk.

3.2 Access and Reception

Patients and consumer organizations are often heard to complain about the difficulty patients have in getting an appointment to see their doctor; in getting to the surgery or health centre (particularly in rural areas); in persuading a doctor to visit at home; and of the brusque manner of some receptionists. Yet when the National Consumer Council did a survey for the Royal Commission on the National Health Service (H.M.S.O., 1979) the general level of satisfaction was high, though some of the anecdotes did not sound quite so favourable.

Communication across a reception hatch or counter is notoriously difficult in any situation. The design of the counter and the need for privacy are important factors. More important is the training and management of receptionists (Drury, 1982).

3.3 Doctor-initiated Communication

General practitioners must decide whether they see their role simply as responding to demand for their services, or whether they try to seek out unmet need, to educate their patients, and to carry out active programmes of surveillance of chronic illness and prevention. In the latter case the doctor must take the initiative and the patient is expected to respond. Many patients do not see this as the general practitioner's proper role, and he may get a hostile response.

What sort of communication does the general practitioner initiate? At its simplest he can write to the patient who has missed an antenatal appointment, or he can inform patients of X-ray and laboratory results. Many practices have handouts for new patients to help them to settle in, and learn how to obtain the services of their new doctor, health visitor, practice nurse etc. This can be a factual list, or can be supplemented by a friendly letter of welcome and perhaps a health questionnaire to form a data-base until the medical record arrives. An early suggestion from the PPG in the author's practice was to have a handout of 'Hints on keeping well" to be widely distributed. It was an opportunity for patients to learn about their doctor's foibles, as well as an encouragement to see health as their own responsibility. The Health Education Council now have excellent booklets on "Looking After Yourself" and "Children's Ailments" which follow the same line. Patients tend to see this policy as evidence of concern, and this encourages their belief that their new surgery or health centre is a friendly place to visit.

This feeling of welcome to a strange waiting room is not helped by a display of imperative posters usually with a negative message "Don't call the doctor out unnecessarily", "Don't bother the doctor with trivial ailments", "Don't be late for your appointment" and so on. The patient who is anxious and uncertain could easily be made to feel that he had no business to be there at all!

Recall systems, surveillance of chronic illness, screening and preventative services all need an efficient information and records system. They also need the co-operation of patients, which can be more easily obtained if they have been consulted when the service is being planned.

Health education is the major professional concern of the health visitor, but the general practitioner is "intervening educationally" (R.C.G.P., 1972) in nearly every consultation. Do they work together? Does the doctor play his full part outside the consulting room to ensure maximum prevention of ill-health? If he does not, it will not be long before he is overwhelmed by increasing demand—for example from an ageing population. Education is the chief weapon in bringing about changes in behaviour. Not all health education is cost-effective, but the influence of the general practitioner talking to his own patients should not be ignored.

3.4 The Patient Participation Group (PPG)

This new development is the main topic of this chapter and will be considered in more detail in later sections.

3.5 The Community Health Council (CHC)

CHCs were established in 1975 in order to provide the patient's viewpoint in planning of the National Health Service. They have not been an instant success, which is not surprising in so unique an experiment. Their responsibilities include the whole field of health care of a population of about a quarter of a million. CHC members regularly visit practices as a "patient's advocate". In most cases they are made welcome and some CHCs have pioneered schemes to help with transport to health centres etc. They also help patients who wish to complain, and that role has not always been popular with G.P.s! Their links with patient opinion are tenuous and it is difficult for them to know where the patients' interests really lie.

Some CHCs have welcomed patient participation groups, and have found in them a useful source of grass-roots information which they badly needed.

3.6 Organizations Operating Mainly at National Level

3.6.1 *Disease/disability Groups*

Some organizations work better if they are centralized at national level, and this applies in particular to the highly specialized disease/disability groups which call on national expertise. They provide communication between specialists, and patients with say—Multiple Sclerosis—or their relatives. They may have local branches, and links with local doctors, but their strength lies in their specialized knowledge and their collective action.

They have proved very successful and their number has multiplied. A recent publication (*General Practitioner*—In Practice Supplement No. 7, 1979) listed 86 diagnostic categories, and over 300 organizations concerned with disability, handicap and mutual help with health problems. They are too numerous for all to be represented at CHC or PPG level.

3.6.2 *Consumer and Community Organizations*

The last decade has seen an increase in the power and influence of consumer organizations. These cover a wide spectrum of interest and activity, much of it outside the health field (e.g. The National Consumer Council, and the Consumers' Association). Some are more specifically concerned with health topics (The National Association of CHCs and the Patients' Association). They are all concerned with the collection of patients' views about services received, and bringing these to the attention of the providers of services. The National Consumer Council has drawn up a "Patient's Charter" to clarify and if necessary improve upon patients' right to care (NCC, 1982). The Consumers' Association (1974–1979) has produced a number of excellent campaign reports and *Which?* reports showing that patients want more of a say in the way health services are run, and are not prepared to leave it to the professionals. This is an indication of the climate of opinion to which the development of patient participation has been a response. This will be considered in the next section.

4 THE DEVELOPMENT OF PATIENT PARTICIPATION

Though the first three patient participation groups were set up independently of each other between 1972 and 1974 (R.C.G.P., 1980) at Berinsfield, Aberdare and Bristol, it is likely that many doctors were consulting their patients as a group on a number of issues before 1972.

The logic of this move was expressed unequivocally by Reedy (1970) at a symposium on a group practice at the Royal College of General Practitioners in 1969:

> It is essential to realize that all the families whose personal and corporate health are embodied within the practice are themselves an integral part of the organization and that operational considerations must include the patient group as a functioning and dynamic integer of the whole organization.

The change which occurred around 1972 was the development of a standing committee of patients to communicate with doctors and staff, in place of the previous *ad hoc* arrangements. The three original groups are still in being after eight to ten years, and over 50 groups now exist. Though many of the newer groups modelled their arrangements on previous groups, the diversity is remarkable. Each group is different, in constitution, in methods and often in name. There is some congruence of aims of all the groups and this will be considered in the next section. The communities served are dissimilar— some being predominantly working-class, some middle-class, and many a mixture of social classes. Each community has its own problems which the PPGs and staff respond to in their separate ways.

The names of the groups differ widely, but all come under the general title of "Patient Participation" (and there is now a National Association for Patient Participation). Several groups reject the idea of having "Patient" in the title for various reasons, such as the broader objectives of the group, the lack of appeal

Table 11.2 Characteristics of patient participation.

1. Patient participation takes place between general practitioners and other primary health care staff on the one hand, and a *group* of interested patients on the other hand.
2. It is a planned and continuing *activity*.
3. The group of patients should be as representative of the population served by the practice as is feasible.
4. The activity is based on the individual practice or health centre.
5. Many activities may be included in patient participation, in response to the varied circumstances of each practice, the different populations served and the individuals who provide care. The following are some examples:
    (a) Helping to shape the aims of the practice, so that some balance is achieved between the aims of the providers and of the users.
    (b) Providing feedback for evaluating current services and planning new ones.
    (c) Calling attention to the needs of community groups which are not being adequately met.
    (d) Using their links with other community agencies to improve the coordination and effectiveness of care.
    (e) Providing a forum for grumbles and complaints—and even praise—by users and providers.
    (f) Helping to develop programmes of prevention which aim to be appropriate to people's health beliefs and level of understanding.
    (g) Working jointly with professional staff to promote health, not just treat sickness, and in so doing to contribute much skill and energy.
    (h) Influencing organizations outside general practice to maintain and improve services.

of the word and its implication of dependent status. In the presence of such diversity, any definition of patient participation is difficult, but an attempt is made in Table 11.2 to list its chief characteristics.

5 FUNCTIONS AND AIMS OF PATIENT PARTICIPATION

The aims of many patient participation groups have not been clearly stated, and these have to be inferred from the activities and functions which develop. Many have been unwilling to state their activities too precisely for fear that this may limit their adaptability. They have clung firmly to their approach of "suck it and see".

Nonetheless there has been a lot in common between the way different PPGs have functioned, and these can be grouped broadly as: feedback; education; safety valve; social support. These four main functions will now be considered in more detail.

5.1 Feedback for Planning and Evaluation

Two of the first three PPGs arose because general practitioners felt the need for feedback from patients in a milieu of change (Paine, 1974; Pritchard, 1975).

The need for an input from patients was seen to be more pressing as general practitioners widened their field of interest towards prevention and responding to need rather than concerning themselves solely with responding to demand from their patients. General practitioners have a clear mandate, deeply rooted in history, to respond to patient's wishes. The mandate to mount screening and surveillance programmes and undertake health education programmes is less clear (Metcalfe, 1980)—one way to obtain such a mandate, which will at the same time improve the planning process, is to obtain an input from patients both at the planning and at the evaluation stages. Joint planning releases a store of knowledge and energy from patients which has resulted in the development of new ways of meeting perceived need. Not only do PPGs produce information—they act upon it. To consult patients in this way helps to lessen the distance between patients as consumers and doctors as decision-makers. There is an analogy between the doctor behaving as a counsellor (listening to the patient, and encouraging him to suggest solutions) in the individual consultation, and similar behaviour in the PPG concerned with different issues. Though the behavioural style has similarities, in the former case the general practitioner fulfils his "doctor" role, in the latter case his role as "manager".

Some doctors do not accept that they have a managerial role, and feel that good rapport with patients in the consultation will solve the problems of providing care without further input from patients. This is a common view among doctors who do not have experience of a PPG. Those with such experience find the feedback from patients useful, constructive and not threatening (Wood and Metcalfe, 1980). Hannay in his study of the "Symptom Iceberg" has demonstrated the alarming extent to which patients needing medical care do not apply for it (Hannay, 1979, 1980). Should primary health care be more responsive to this unexpressed need, and modify its services accordingly? As Hannay reminds us "any system without a feedback loop runs wild". This input from patients is available also to influence the provision of services outside primary care, such as hospital or social services. By its closeness to the point of delivery of the service, the combined feedback from several PPGs in a district might have an advantage over existing sources of information to health authorities from community health councils, from lay members and from pressure groups.

Another function of the PPG is to ensure that the primary health care staff are aware of the real life situation in the community they serve. This is particularly important when the staff live outside the practice area. Many of the issues (e.g. unemployment, poor housing, poverty, population shift and other social disadvantages) are likely to be well known to all members of the primary health care team from their daily contacts, but the effect of a PPG is to give an extra dimension to this feeling of community; to bridge the knowledge and attitude gap, and to make planning more realistic and the service more responsive.

5.2 Education

Health education is the main activity of some groups. The Aberdare PPG (Wilson, 1975) has pioneered this approach. It has organized over 140 public lectures and has made films and video tapes to explain health problems in terms the local population can understand, and to encourage healthy living and the prevention of illness. Though the lecturers are likely to be experts, the arrangement of the programme is in the hands of the patients' committee. These lectures bring the PPG to the notice of those attending, and so encourage participation in other fields.

A different experiment has been tried in an area with high patient turnover at Kentish Town in North London. A rota of patients do duty in the waiting room to bring the available services to the notice of newly-arrived patients. They are helped by audio-visual displays. These volunteers have links with other community networks and agencies, and so make the health centre the focus for a wide range of help. They can also bring complaints and suggestions to the notice of staff, and can monitor waiting times and patient satisfaction. They also discovered that some people only came to read the magazines or pass the time, with no intention of seeing the doctor!

Another experiment at Glyncorrwg in South Wales is to have a medical library for patients in the waiting room. This is a predominantly working-class area, and the library has proved popular. This helps to dispel the myth that it is only the middle-class patients who are interested in health topics.

Education is a two-way process, and it is important that doctors and staff should be involved in these activities so that they can learn more about the health needs and aspirations of the community they serve, with the aim of making the service more effective.

5.3 A Safety Valve

No service is perfect, and the primary care service is bound to generate its share of complaints. But how can complaints best be aired and answered? Patients have always been reluctant to complain, particularly if they are receiving medical treatment. They need to feel strongly in order to overcome this reluctance. Usually the aim is to save it happening to someone else, rather than to exact punishment or damages.

In general the sooner a complaint can be brought to the point at which it occurred the better. Once time passes, and the bureaucratic complaints procedure grinds into action, defensive positions are taken up, and adaptive communication stops. PPGs deal mostly with general complaints. Some have a panel to help with individual complaints. This mechanism has the advantage of interposing a neutral link-person between the complaining patient and the doctor. Mostly these panels seem to work satisfactorily. There is no firm evidence that formal complaints are fewer where there is this informal safety valve, but CHC members have stated that practices with PPGs generate very few complaints. This is to be expected, as Wood and Metcalfe (1980) have shown that practices with PPGs are not typical. Short of the need for complaint, patients see the service from their viewpoint, and are good at making constructive suggestions. A suggestion box will pick up a few, but general discussion in a PPG results in practical improvements in the service. Patients feel that their suggestions are acted upon (where possible) or are discussed in a reasonable adult-to-adult manner. It comes as a pleasant surprise to many patients to be able to have an equal sort of dialogue with doctors and staff, particularly so where there is a class or culture barrier to surmount. Doctors in the consultation may do their best to cast aside the traditional parent–child relationship, but this is not always possible because the patient is anxious and perhaps ill, and the doctor is the fount of knowledge and healing! Away from the medical setting this disparity can disappear, particularly when the patient's knowledge and energy is being used to suggest and help provide an improved service.

Patients with experience of a PPG say that the doctor becomes more approachable, and this leads to an increase of respect, but less awe. Does this lessening of "distance" decrease the doctor's power? It may act as a brake on the abuse of power, but there is no detectable shift of power, and the combined power of staff and patients working in concert is increased *vis-à-vis* outside agencies. There are numerous examples of this, where authorities do not respond to requests from doctors, but do respond to requests from PPGs (e.g. in keeping an ambulance station or outpatient service open). Maybe this is because the views of local groups of patients are valued more because they are hard to get, whereas doctors' views are less so. This suggests the possibility that PPGs are manipulated by the doctors who form them. There is little doubt that this is possible, and may happen on occasions where the action of a PPG meets the doctors' objectives but not necessarily those of the patients, which is nothing to be ashamed of if it is done openly. It must be balanced by a trade-off in which the doctor goes along with patients' objectives, even at the expense of his own interests. Unless there is some balance of advantage to staff and patients the group is not likely to remain active.

One effect of an open dialogue is to expose the anxieties which patients have about the secrecy surrounding case notes, letters to consultants and side-effects of drugs. The logical step is that this leads to more "open" medicine and explanation. Some doctors may feel that they are giving away trade secrets and lessening their professional status. In these times when professional knowledge of all kinds is not held in very high esteem and exclusivity is frowned upon, the advantage of sharing knowledge far outweighs the danger. The doctor who refuses to share this knowledge can often be by-passed by resort to public libraries or phone-in radio programmes.

It has been suggested that PPGs are a sort of "social audit", and the G.P. and staff are made more accountable to a group of their patients. In my view this is true, in just the same way as medical audit leads to more accountability in technical matters. This may offend some doctors (as does medical audit) but it is as well to ponder on the alternative. Politicians, and those professionals and administrators who do not enjoy the G.P.s' freedom from managerial restraints are keen to limit this freedom by bureaucratic intervention. In my view it is preferable that a G.P. should be accountable to his patients, rather than to a bureaucracy which does not understand the sort of risk-business which is primary health care. Patients understand it far better.

General practitioners and other staff work under great pressure: they too need a safety valve which the regulations do not provide. They can sound off to their peers or spouses, but a mature PPG can understand some of the general practitioner's problems and frustrations in providing care, and allow the opportunity for their expression and amelioration (Hillier, 1980).

5.4 Social Support Services

At a time when medicine is becoming more technical and social services have greatly expanded it might be expected that the pastoral and social activity of the primary health care team would decrease. There are two reasons why this might not be so. First, that needs vary greatly between neighbourhoods—even between different parts of one practice—so that centralized services operating on "norms of provision" cannot easily take account of local differences. Secondly, it is well known that different local authorities provide different levels and standards of service, depending on their resources and their philosophy.

It was therefore natural that some PPGs, notably Bristol (Paine, 1974; Dakin and Milligan, 1980) should uncover the need for certain social support activities (e.g. luncheon clubs for the elderly, transport services for the infirm, postnatal support groups etc.) and fill the need from their own resources, based on the health centre. This has an enormous advantage for general practitioners and staff who have a wide range of services available for their patients without a referral barrier. Patients benefit too by being helped by other patients of the practice rather than by professional social agencies. Many patients (particularly the elderly) refuse professional help because they feel that it carries the stigma of accepting charity. This is less likely to happen if patient helps patient, and the person helped may later contribute as a helper.

In my own practice voluntary drivers have been bringing patients to the surgery or health centre for over 15 years without missing a day. The drivers insist on paying for their own petrol as their contribution, in which they take great pride. This contribution which patients make to the work of the doctor may improve their relationship so that it is nearer to reciprocity, rather than the doctor providing medical care as a gift to the patient.

6 IMPLICATIONS FOR RESEARCH AND EDUCATION

6.1 Research

The field of research into patient–doctor communication outside the consulting room is too large to be considered in this chapter, and is far beyond my competence. I will therefore consider research into patient participation primarily.

The first papers (Paine, 1974; Pritchard, 1975; Wilson, 1975)—all by general practitioners—described the first three PPGs and attempted to discuss their effectiveness for patient care, without any attempt at evaluation of outcome. The next group of papers (Sand, 1978, 1980; Shaw, 1978; Graffy, 1979, 1980; Davies, 1979; Wood and Metcalfe, 1980) were by researchers outside patient participation who studied from one to fifteen groups and made critical assessments of their value. These should be studied in the original as only a few salient points can be mentioned here.

The first to appear was the thesis by Peter Sand (1978) head of research of the Consumer Association. He sent questionnaires to members of four PPGs, studied their minutes and visited the practices. He noted the enthusiasm of the groups, and analysed their composition, and the other interests of members. He thought that transfer of power was an unlikely outcome. He noted that only a small number of the patient population were involved, that complaints were a minor preoccupation, and that the groups he studied were dependent on the enthusiasm of the doctors. He thought PPGs were of value to CHCs in improving consumer representation in health services generally, and listed some of their solid achievements in improving the organization of care programmes and in health education. The more nebulous area of doctor–patient communication was difficult to evaluate objectively, but was seen as a fundamental goal of PPGs.

The next study by Shaw (1978) for the Welsh Consumer Council focused on one group (Aberdare). His study of patient's committee members had broadly the same conclusions as Sand's. He also interviewed 37 patients who consented out of 80 who attended the health centre on one day. Twenty-five had heard of the committee, eight were regarded as fairly well informed about their activities, and 12 expressed willingness to join the committee. Both patients and doctors thought that the committee should consist of ordinary citizens motivated by high ideals and not having specialized knowledge. There is detailed discussion of accountability and "open medicine".

The studies of Graffy (1979, 1980) and Davies (1979), each of six PPGs, covered similar ground and reached similar conclusions to Sand's. The level of discussion in both these papers—by medical students—is extremely high. Accurate descriptive studies of this kind are extremely valuable as a base for designing and carrying out evaluative studies.

Wood and Metcalfe (1980) in a telephone survey questioned 14 lay members and ten general practitioners from 15 PPGs. They classified the four main categories of activity (feedback, education, safety valve, social support) which I have used in Section 5. They further divided the activities into:

(a) Practice-oriented activities—giving patients a say—dealing with complaints;

(b) Practice-neighbourhood links—strengthening bonds between staff and patients, and with other neighbourhood networks;

(c) Neighbourhood-oriented activities—encouragement of self-care—change in other parts of N.H.S.

The doctors who had formed PPGs did not conform to any stereotype, but tended to be "counsellors" or "moderns" rather than "technicians" or "withdrawers" (Mechanic, 1975). Lay members of the groups were constructive in their approach rather than complaining.

A further telephone survey was done of 15 general practitioner trainers who did not have PPGs. Five had heard of them. The contrary views of those with experience of PPGs and the 15 trainers is summarized in Table 11.3.

Table 11.3.

24 with experience of PPGs	15 trainers without experience of PPGs
Reduce friction	increase friction
Increase understanding	unnecessary
Improve effectiveness	decrease effectiveness
Extend role	limit role
An essential tool	a current fad

Evaluation of achievement of objectives has not been undertaken by PPGs to any great extent. This is perhaps surprising as many PPGs have been formed to help evaluate patient care, but have not taken the next logical step of evaluating the PPG.

Some PPGs have clearly stated objectives from which some outcome might be derived and evaluated: others do not state their objectives, which can only be inferred from the nature of their activities.

This evaluation by PPGs themselves (with outside help) of their achievements is, in my opinion, the next step to be taken if credibility is sought. A controlled study of similar practices with and without PPGs would be valuable but with so many variables it would have to be a large and detailed study. Such a study has been planned (Wood, 1980a) using qualitative rather than quantitative assessment.

6.2 Education

Vocational training for general practice has tended to concentrate on the one-to-one consultation as the norm (RCGP, 1972). Team working, group therapy and health education all require a different style of communication for which doctors have had little or no training. (Clinical psychologists, health visitors and community social workers may be skilled in one or more of these three areas.) Is a special skill needed for general practitioners who are involved in PPGs? If so could this be defined and taught? There are signs that social skills training will be available for some general practitioners. It is hoped that this training will cover team working and PPGs in their remit.

The support and enthusiasm of general practitioners is needed if PPGs are to succeed. If patient participation is to be encouraged, then educational effort must concentrate on G.P.s. A start was made on the 16th January, 1980, with a study day at the Royal College of General Practitioners. Sixty-eight general practitioners, five patient representatives, four social scientists and 14 from the press and media attended. The President of the College (Dr John Horder) took the chair. Demand for places was such that 50 more general practitioners applied than could be included.

The study day was evaluated by questionnaires, one completed beforehand and the other after a lapse of three months (Wood, 1980b). Of 26 responding doctors who did not previously have a group in their practice, seven had formed a group and 16 were taking positive action to form one. Three were opposed to the idea. All those who had formed a group had considered it before attending the study day. It was not possible to measure the part played by the study day in encouraging the formation of groups, but the general impression of participants was favourable.

7 IN CONCLUSION

Is patient participation an essential part of general practice or just a happy hunting ground for enthusiasts? The same question might be asked about team working, medical audit or health education. All these topics represent a shift of the doctor's role from the one-to-one consultation into a wider role. It represents an opportunity and a threat. If the "doctor" strays into being a "manager" will this reinforce or diminish his essential "doctor" role? These and many other questions remain to be answered, but those general practitioners and patients who have experience of a PPG see clear benefits arising from it.

In my view it is a normative and adaptive mechanism which helps general practice to meet change and increase its effectiveness. If successful, it should benefit patient–doctor communication at all levels and by whatever pathway it occurs.

ACKNOWLEDGEMENTS

I wish to thank many people on whose ideas I have freely drawn, and who have helped with comments on the manuscript, but in particular Anna Ford, Sheila Hillier, Joan Mant, David Metcalfe, Wendy Pritchard, Barry Reedy and Jo Wood. I wish also to thank all those patients whose contribution made it all happen.

REFERENCES

Consumers' Association (1974–1979). *Which?* report *"Doctors"*, January 1974. Campaign reports: "Managing at home", August 1978; "Treating medical complaints", October 1978; "Registering with a doctor", January 1979. The Consumers' Association, 14 Buckingham Street, London WC2N 6DS.

Dakin, A. and Milligan, J. (1980). The patient's point of view. Patient participation. *J. Roy. Coll. Gen. Pract.* **30**, 133–135; and in R.C.G.P. (1981).

Davies, A. (1979). Dissertation on Patient Participation. Bedford College, University of London.

Drury, M. (1982). *The Medical Secretary and Receptionist's Handbook*, 4th edn. Baillière-Tindall, London.

General Practitioner (1979). In Practice Supplement No. 7 to General Practitioner, 19 October 1979. Haymarket Press, London.

Graffy, J. (1979). Dissertation on Patient Participation. University of Birmingham.

Graffy, J. (1980). Patient participation in primary health care. *J. Roy. Coll. Gen. Pract.* **30**, 542–545.

Hannay, D. (1979). *The Symptom Iceberg. A Study of Community Health.* Routledge & Kegan Paul, London.

Hannay, D. (1980). The "iceberg" of illness and "trivial" consultations. *J. Roy. Coll. Gen. Pract.* **30**, 551–554.

Health Education Council (1980). "Advice to Patients" by Professor David Morrell. "Looking after Yourself" by Dr. Alan Maryon Davis.

Hillier, S. (1980). Can patients influence decisions about health care? Paper given at Royal College of General Practitioners study day 16 January 1980. See R.C.G.P. (1981).

H.M.S.O. (1979). *Access to Primary Care.* Royal Commission on the Health Service, London.

Last, J. M. (1967). Objective measurements of quality in General Practice. Supplement to *Ann. Gen. Pract. XII*, 2.

Mechanic, D. (1975). Practice orientation among general practitioners in England and Wales. In *A Sociology of Medical Practice* (O. Cox and A. Mead, ed.). Collier-Macmillan, London.

Metcalfe, D. (1980). The role of patient participation in the development of rational health services. Paper given at Royal College of General Practitioners study day 16 January 1980. See R.C.G.P. (1981).

N.C.C. (1982). *Patients' Rights. A Guide to the Responsibilities of Patients and Doctors in the NHS.* National Consumer Council, London.

Paine, T. F. (1974). Patient's association in general practice. *J. Roy. Coll. Gen. Pract.* **24**, 351.

Pritchard, P. (1975). Community participation in primary health care. *Br. Med. J.* 2, 583.

Pritchard, P. (1979). Patient Participation in Primary Health Care. *Health Trends* 11, 92–95. H.M.S.O. London.

Pritchard, P. (1980). Study day on patient participation *J. Roy. Coll. Gen. Pract.* 30, 250–252.

Pritchard, P. (1981). *Manual of Primary Health Care*, 2nd edn. Oxford University Press, Oxford.

R.C.G.P. (1972). The future general practitioner. Learning and teaching. *Roy. Coll. Gen. Pract. Brit. Med. J.* London.

R.C.G.P. (1978). Birmingham Research Unit. Practice activity analysis. Referral rates. *J. Roy. Coll. Gen. Pract.* 28. 60.

R.C.G.P. (1980) Patient participation. Editorial. *J. Roy. Coll. Gen. Pract.* 30, 132.

R.C.G.P. (1981). *Patient Participation in General Practice* (P. Pritchard, ed.) Occasional Paper No. 17. Royal College of General Practitioners, London.

Reedy, B. (1970). Operational problems in group practice. *J. Roy. Coll. Gen. Pract.* 20, Supp. No. 2, p. 72.

Robinson, D. (1978). *Patients, Practitioners and Medical Care*, 2nd edn. Heinemann, London.

Sand, P. (1978). Patient participation in general practice. A research study. MSc. Thesis. University of Surrey. Guildford.

Sand, P. (1980). *Patient Participation in General Practice* . See R.C.G.P. (1981).

Shaw, I. (1978). *Patient Participation in General Practice.* Welsh Consumer Council, Cardiff.

Suchman. (1965). Stages of illness and medical care. *J. Hlth Hum. Behav.* 6, 114.

Wilson, A. (1975). Participation by patients in primary care. *J. Roy. Coll. Gen. Pract.* 25, 906.

Wood, J. (1980a). Personal communication.

Wood, J. (1980b). The impact of the study day held at Royal College of General Practitioners on 16 January 1980. See R.C.G.P. (1981).

Wood, J. and Metcalfe, D. (1980). Professional attitudes to patient participation groups: an exploratory study. *J. Roy. Coll. Gen. Pract.* 30, 538–541 (and in R.C.A.P. (1981)).

Wright, H. J. (1978). The aetiology of consultation. *J. Roy. Coll. Gen. Pract.* 28, 400.

Part IV
Medical Education and Medical Practice

12   The Mismatch between Undergraduate Education and the Medical Task

David Metcalfe

It has been said that the search for an ideal medical school curriculum is like the search for the Holy Grail. In remembering the other preoccupations of the "questing knight" one is reminded that the search for the mythical beast was facilitated by the collection and analysis of its droppings, or "fewmets". The study of the products of conventional medical education may be more illuminating than a consideration of its entrails and in some ways more productive!

The immediate product of undergraduate medical education is the "junior doctor" or intern, and he or she has a job to do which is largely defined by the immediate needs of the patients to whose care he or she contributes in no small part. Just as "the child is father to the man" it seems reasonable to suppose that the "set" of knowledge, skills, attitudes, and hence behaviour of the junior doctor will, unless something extraordinary occurs, predict certain aspects of his or her behaviour throughout a lifetime in practice of "the art so long to learn". Shortcomings in that behaviour which are likely to be persistent must be related either to the people selected for medical education, or to the process of that education, or both. That there are such shortcomings (despite, in every Western Society, the fact that medical schools can pick and choose an elite from a large number of suitably qualified applicants) is attested to by much anecdote and some formal research, and should motivate medical educators to anxious introspection!

Junior doctors are thought to be over-dependent on, and indiscriminate in their selection of, diagnostic investigations, and unwilling to rely on their basic clinical skills of history taking and physical examination.

This may be related to their poor communication skills with patients, which in turn has been shown not only to result in patient dissatisfaction and distress, but also in faulty diagnosis.

In any case, their efforts at diagnosis often demonstrate a poor grasp of probability.

In those situations in which they have responsibility for selection of medication they tend to prescribe expensive, complex and under-evaluated drugs rather than cheap, well-understood and well-used medicaments. They are not well-equipped to evaluate the evidence for the efficacy and safety of new drugs.

They are similarly not well-equipped to cope with their patients' distress, anxiety, or even their need for comprehensible information, and are seen by patients as lacking in the caring qualities.

These shortcomings can, and do, lead to behaviour that transgresses the ethical imperative of primacy for the patients safety, autonomy, dignity and comfort: a very senior professor of medicine has said he is "appalled at what is done *to* patients for publication and promotion rather than their own good".

Lastly, the well recognized hiatus in learning habits of the intern year (and who can blame the young doctor, with Finals passed, expected to work a 70–100 hour week?) may be self-perpetuating, or at any rate self-repeating once examinations necessary for promotion are passed.

Of course, very few graduates exhibit all these shortcomings, and some seem to avoid all. Nevertheless, each one is prevalent enough to cause concern, particularly to the consultants on whose units they serve. Curiously these self same specialists, who bewail the "manifold sins and wickednesses" of their house staff, if challenged, rally to their defence in general terms: "But really, all things considered, they're remarkably good. . . !" What then, are the "all things" that should be considered?

First, the learning experience of these young doctors has been clouded by five unresolved issues which either continue to plague those charged with designing their curricula, or have been resolutely expunged from that design process.

The first of these is the old debate "education or training": learning for its own sake, or learning to do a job. Apart from the fact that most medical education is paid for, wholly or in part, by Governments, in order to staff their Health Services, and that those governments would consider such debate arcane if not downright irresponsible, the difference is probably, nowadays, unreal. Both share the basic principle of providing knowledge as a basis for clear thinking (or problem solving): the debate is about the relevance of the knowledge provided.

Accordingly, the second issue concerns whether subjects should be taught "as the pure discipline" or "as applied to medicine". Students are particularly sceptical of the behavioural sciences when taught as subjects "in their own right", but could profitably address their sceptism to much of the bio-chemistry and some of the anatomy to which they are subjected. Assurance of relevance in such subjects is, of course threatened, even where it is sought, by the ever decreasing number of clinically qualified (let alone experienced) members of staff in such departments.

Another issue is the balance of teaching between "diagnosis" and "management": most students feel that 80% of their learning time is spent on the former, and only 20% on the latter. Easily explicable as this distribution of educational effort may be, it enshrines diagnosis as the acme of intellectual activity, rather than effective, efficient and patient centred management, which must, after all be the objective of medical care. (Of course diagnosis is a crucial step in management, but a moment's reflection reveals than in some acute crisis situations management precedes the precise definition of the pathophysiology; that in the care of chronic diseases the diagnosis may be far in the past, but the management decision is today; and lastly that the vast majority of doctor–patient interactions are "follow-ups", and therefore management directed rather than diagnosis directed.)

The fourth unresolved issue is how to provide the student with an appropriate understanding of the relative positions of "curing" and "caring" in the medical task. As the acute infections recede into the background as major components of the medical task (thanks not only to antibiotics and asepsis, but even more to public health and preventive medicine) the control of irreversible pathophysiology and alleviation of disability and handicap emerge as the prime concern of the clinician. The student is seldom helped to adjust, from his or her youthful idealism, to the reality: most of the major diseases that we encounter are incurable when first diagnosed. This failure compounds the diagnosis/management issue: the diagnosis having been made, the student feels, there is nothing much more to be done by the clinician!

If the foregoing unresolved issues have been those of "objectives" and "content", the last concerns "method", and centres on examinations. The conflict between examinations which are relevant to the task and, of themselves, learning opportunities, and those which are technically more reliable and administratively more practicable has been largely resolved, under pressure of student numbers in favour of the latter. The intellectual activity required by essays, vivas, and clinical exams appear significantly different from that by MCQs. It is interesting to note that students *"post mortems"* on the former check facts and rehearse arguments put forward: on the latter, all that is exchanged is the number of questions answered! What you know is more important than what you don't know! From what is known of the relationship between student learning and examinations, such an issue has major impli-cations.

Not only, however, is the student the victim of unresolved issues: his or her learning opportunities in the clinical course are often significantly affected by circumstances which did not apply to the clinical training of those who now design and administer the curriculum. Today's students suffer viccissitudes to do with grants, housing and travel that few of today's senior clinical teachers experienced. But apart from such "domestic" matters, there are other handicaps. Students often feel that nursing staff are anything from unhelpful to downright hostile (and it is easy to forget the evolving professionalism of nurses away from the "clinical handmaiden" stereotype, means that medical students' education occupies a lowly place on the nursing agenda, being sometimes, especially in midwifery, directly in competition). The shortness of inpatient stays, and the intensity of diagnostic/therapeutic activity during them makes it difficult for the student to "get at the patients" at all (they are always up at X-ray, down in physio, having special tests, or in the bath!) let alone do so in a relaxed and patient way that would enhance his or her interpersonal skills. It is seldom possible for a student to follow-up a patient closely enough to establish, in his or her mind, the "natural history" even of the hospital phase of the illness. In any case today's students frequently express concern, hesitation, or even repugnance, for "using sick people to learn on", yet are seldom given a role, *vis-à-vis* the patient, that they can see as contributing to his or her wellbeing. Meanwhile the hospital morbidity, whether in terms of age, or diagnostic mix is less and less representative of the morbidity (or need) of the community in which it is situated. Many older clinicians will remember the central place in their learning occupied by TB and neurosyphilis, conditions which had largely disappeared in the population even then, let alone when they emerged into independent practice! One of the learning opportunities conferred by the preponderance of chronic degenerative disease is the dependence of long-term care on good clinical records. Yet on most units, such records are not kept, let alone used for teaching!

The education that we provide for our students therefore is affected by unresolved issues and unplanned handicaps. These result in a significant mismatch between the pattern of undergraduate learning and the graduates' task. This mismatch may pertain not only to the few years after graduation, but even longer into the developing career of the young doctor. To some extent this mismatch is the result of the factors so far discussed, and to some extent independent of them. There are six cardinal discrepancies.

First, the use of high grades in scientific subjects as a criterion for entry selects people who do most of their thinking in a "convergent" mode: the problem solving approach in clinical medicine is best served by "divergent" thinking.

This selection bias is compounded by the use of inductive problem solving in the preclinical and early clinical course: it has been shown that clinicians formulate hypotheses very early in the transaction and use a hypothetical-deductive problem solving routine. The student is neither advised or helped to make the transition.

In the preclinical subjects the student is taught *on* inanimate learning materials (laboratory equipment, slides, "pots", cadavers, and post-mortem material) and on the wards the teaching is again *on* undressed, horizontal and largely non-autonomous patients). Indeed patients are often described by teaching consultants as "clinical material" (as in "I haven't got very good material on my ward this week!"). The essence of medical practice is that the doctor works *with* patients whose autonomy is, most of the time intact, and he should be concerned to *preserve* it.

Of course, the main learning environment is the ward which is, or appears to the student at any rate, a doctor controlled environment, yet the large majority of medical care, specialist and generalist, is undertaken in the patients' environment which is certainly not doctor controlled!

Fifthly, the student is taught in "high certainty areas" not only in the basic sciences, but in the wards of teaching hospitals (Flexner's concept of excellence has become synonymous with precision), yet much of clinical practice requires logical decision making in low certainty areas.

Lastly, the students' learning is conditioned by anxiety, not only from examination pressure but also by the idiom of much clinical teaching. (As Freeling pointed out, many of our aphorisms inculcate anxiety: "if you don't do this . . . that will happen. If you don't put your finger in it you will put your foot in it" etc.) Clinical practice however requires calm not only for better decision making, but for transmission to patients.

Given then, that the graduates find these major disparities between the way they learned and the way they are expected to function, what is the likely result? They clearly recognize the conflict (which of course adds to the strains of the intern year) and this generates considerable anxiety as to whether they are competent (and feelings of guilt if they feel that they are not). They have, therefore, to erect and operate a "coping strategy". In most cases this will be one of acceptance, tinged with anger directed toward those who were responsible for their medical education, and a determination to learn, in their own way, to do the job properly. These young doctors can be expected to grow, and to progress towards the appropriate behaviours: they are the survivors! In a significant minority, however, the coping strategy adopted is one of "denial" (that they feel inadequate) and therefore they need rigidly to control the situation in order to contain the uncertainty and perplexity inherent in their clinical role. One can well hear them say "Lets do some more tests to sort this out"; "I've got a diagnosis: don't knock mine (however far fetched) till you have a better one"; "Of course I prescribed X: someone told me it was very good and I haven't got time to evaluate it myself"; and, to a patient, explicitly or implicitly "Don't open up problem areas I can't cope with, like your feelings—I've got problems of my own".

If these are the "fewmets", the mythical beast is in need of treatment.

13 Communication Skills Training in United Kingdom Medical Schools

Richard Wakeford

1 INTRODUCTION

The aim of this chapter is to review the place of communication skills training in undergraduate medical schools in the United Kingdom, and to contrast the situation briefly with that in the U.S.A. The effect of a communication skills training programme is then discussed, and one experiment reported in detail. Finally, the difficulty of introducing the subject into medical schools' curricula is reviewed in an attempt to identify obstacles to change in medical education in the U.K. generally.

The size of the ultimate problem—that of doctors, many of whom are unable to communicate efficiently with their patients and colleagues—has been well documented. Chapter 4 by Ley in this volume has demonstrated serious communication failures between doctors and their patients, leading to such undesirable outcomes as an average of less than 50% compliance with medical advice. Junek *et al.* (1979) found that interviewing skills amongst psychiatric residents were inadequate and needed to be enhanced. Segall and Roberts (1980) report that doctors' estimates of patients' understanding of medical terminology are far from good; indeed, the words which doctors use between themselves to communicate levels of uncertainty or certainty are very variable in their intended meanings as described by Bryant and Norman (1979). Fletcher (1979) in an important review of the teaching of communication skills, concludes that "the main consequence of faulty interviewing must be inadequate or even wrong diagnosis leading to wrong treatment. The commonest error is diagnosis of physical disease when the real problem is psycho-social". The result, as Ley shows, is that the outcome of consultations and medical care is less satisfactory than it might be.

Carroll and Monroe (1979) reviewed a total of 73 studies on the teaching of medical interviewing. They concluded that "the importance of medical interviewing skills is demonstrated by recent research identifying inter-personal communications as a major course of variance in patient satisfaction, patient compliance, and the incidence of malpractice litigation". Indeed, a report in the U.S.A. in *Science News* (1973) has shown that poor communication between physician and patient is now the single most common cause of malpractice suits.

The need for urgent examination of this area of medical education was originally highlighted by Helfer (1970) who demonstrated that students in the first year of medical school performed significantly better on many aspects of the interview than their "trained" colleagues at the end of the medical course. This supports the conclusion of Sir George Pickering (1978), arrived at after a lifetime of work in medical education, that

> my extensive contacts with young doctors in the United Kingdom and the United States have led me to conclude that their greatest single defect is their inability to take a really good history, and to be able to sit down and listen to their patients in such a way that they really learn what the patient's problems are that most deeply trouble him.

2 COMMUNICATION SKILLS TRAINING IN UNDERGRADUATE MEDICAL EDUCATION

2.1 The Position in the United Kingdom

Supervision of basic medical education (undergraduate training plus the pre-registration year) rests with the General Medical Council, established by Act of Parliament in 1858. From time to time, it has issued Recommendations which have governed the form and content of the undergraduate medical curriculum. Up to 1967, these Recommendations were limiting and specific, suggesting for example the number of hours which needed to be devoted to anatomy in the pre-clinical course. Those of 1967 were, however, much more liberal, laying down only the broadest guidelines, and encouraging schools to experiment, diversify and innovate. Following a survey of medical education in the U.K. by the General Medical Council (1977), further Recommendations have been issued, now by the Education Committee of the reorganized Council (1980).

These new Recommendations include a list of objectives for the under-graduate period of training: these are shown in Table 13.1. No fewer than three of these 20 objectives include explicit reference to the skills of communication.

Table 13.1 Objectives of undergraduate medical education in the U.K.

The student should by the time of qualification have sufficient knowledge of the structure and functions of the human body in health and disease, of normal and abnormal human behaviour and of the techniques of diagnosis and treatment, to enable him to assume the responsibilities of a pre-registration House Officer and to prepare him for vocational training for a speciality (including general practice), followed by continuing education throughout his professional career. The graduate's knowledge should thus include the basic principles underlying the subjects which he has been taught but need not include those detailed aspects which are more appropriate to specialized vocational training.

In order to achieve this object, it is necessary for a student

1. To acquire knowledge and understanding of:
   (a) The sciences upon which Medicine depends and the scientific and experimental method;
   (b) The structure, function and normal growth and development of the human body and the workings of the mind and their interaction, the factors which may disturb these, and the disorders of structure and function which may result;
   (c) The aetiology, natural history and prognosis of the common mental and physical ailments. Students must have experience of emergencies and a good knowledge of the commoner disabling diseases, and of ageing processes;
   (d) Normal pregnancy and childbirth, the commoner obstetric emergencies, the principles of ante-natal and post-natal care, and medical aspects of family planning and psycho-sexual counselling;
   (e) The principles of prevention and of therapy, including health education, the amelioration of suffering and disability, rehabilitation, the maintenance of health in old age, and the care of the dying;
   (f) Human relationships, both personal and communal, and the interaction between man and his physical, biological and social environment;
   (g) The organization and provision of health care in the community and in hospital, the identification of the need for it, and the economic, ethical and practical constraints within which it operates; and
   (h) The ethical standards and legal responsibilities of the medical profession.

2. To develop the professional skills necessary:
   (a) To elicit, record and interpret the relevant medical history, symptoms and physical signs, and to identify the problems and how these may be managed;
   (b) To carry out simple practical clinical procedures;
   (c) To deal with common medical emergencies;
   (d) To communicate effectively and sensitively with patients and their relatives;
   (e) To communicate clinical information accurately and concisely, both by word of mouth and in writing, to medical colleagues and to other professionals involved in the care of the patient; and
   (f) To use laboratory and other diagnostic and therapeutic services effectively and economically, and in the best interests of his patient.

3. To develop appropriate attitudes to the practice of Medicine, which include:
   (a) Recognition that a blend of scientific and humanitarian approaches is needed in medicine;
   (b) A capacity for self education, so that he may continue to develop and extend his knowledge and skills throughout his professional life, and recognize his obligation to contribute if he can to the progress of medicine and to new knowledge;

Table 13.1 Objectives of undergraduate medical education in the U.K.—*cont.*

(c) The ability to assess the reliability of evidence and the relevance of scientific knowledge, to reach conclusions by logical deduction or by experiment, and to evaluate critically methods and standards of medical practice;

(d) A continuing concern for the interests and dignity of his patients;

(e) An ability to appreciate the limitations of his own knowledge, combined with a willingness, when necessary, to seek further help; and

(f) The achievement of good working relationships with members of the other health care professions.

It is too soon to see how the medical schools will respond to these more detailed recommendations, but the situation in 1975–77 in the medical schools as far as communication skills training is concerned is well documented—in part by the GMC Survey of Basic Medical Education (1977) and in part by a personal survey by Professor Fletcher (1979). The teaching of communication skills regularly occurred in only three medical schools in the U.K. in the pre-clinical stage of the course. Out of a total of thirty clinical schools, there were nine in which no attempt was made to develop the students' interpersonal skills: of these, there were three or four in which significant senior members of staff such as the Dean or Senior Professor of Medicine were positively against the idea of attempting to teach the subject.

The remaining twenty schools did make some attempt to teach communication skills. Within this number, there were twelve in which departments or units of general practice took it upon themselves to attempt to develop students' interpersonal skills. In eleven schools, including some of the above, departments of psychiatry were active. In addition to these departments, there were two universities with joint departments of community medicine and general practice attempting to develop students' communication skills. In the remaining schools, a variety of idiosyncratic situations obtained: in one, there was a professor of medicine conducting research on the topic; in a second, the paediatricians were working in this area; two departments of surgery made attempts to teach communication skills; and at two further schools, multidisciplinary groups were active.

It is important to note that in only one medical school was there a formal and deliberate decision at central faculty level that communication skills training should form a defined part of the course for all students. In the vast majority of schools in which teaching of the subject was undertaken, it was because interested individuals within departments decided to use some of the time allocated to them for the teaching of this subject rather than other aspects of their speciality. Thus by no means all the students in a school with, for example, an "interested" Professor of Medicine, would receive training in the subject.

The most common teaching method involved video-tape recording. A student is recorded conducting an interview with a patient: this is then played back with him, either singly or in a small group, and reviewed by a teacher. This may be supported by other activities: an example involved a number of students interviewing the same patient, followed by a discussion between students, patient and tutor. Virtually all the teaching concerned the development of students' history-taking skills: with only a single exception, no teaching was discovered on what Fletcher calls the "exposition"—how to give information to patients.

In summary, in 1975–77 approximately one third of British Medical Schools offered no training in communication skills. In the remainder, it was normally provided within the ambit of general practice or psychiatry and amounted to one or two hours of video recording and replay. Not all students in any individual medical school necessarily received the training, except that in one school, it was given to all. There was thus little institutional commitment in U.K. medical schools to the teaching of communication skills—though very recently an enlighted English publisher has produced a brief and stimulating book, the report of a Working Party chaired by Walton (1980), on the subject for medical students and their teachers.

2.2 The Situation in the U.S.A.

A recent paper by Kahn *et al.* (1979) reported a questionnaire survey of U.S. medical schools' teaching of communication skills at about the same time. Just over 70% replied, with 96% of these reporting that they did offer courses on the teaching of interpersonal skills. Thus, between 67% and 96% of American schools taught the subject. In the group of respondents, there were found to be over 500 individual medical school faculty members teaching interpersonal skills to medical students, more than four per school. An average of 2·5 official, school-instituted interpersonal skills programmes were reported per school.

Sixty-one per cent of these courses in the U.S.A. were directed to pre-clinical students, with 26% being offered to clinical students: the remaining 13% spanned both phases of the course. Virtually all the medical schools reported that a principal vehicle for the teaching was video technology. Whilst the heaviest emphasis was on information-gathering, a significant minority of the schools also gave training in the field of information-giving. The survey also identified what were described as "special application areas" in which some schools gave training. Examples were: suicide prevention; sexual counselling; and counselling the deaf and dumb. Indeed, over half of the responding schools specifically attempted to teach students how to work with "difficult" patients. About one third of the schools evaluated the outcome of the programme in some way.

Contrasted with the U.K. situation, there was clearly a very significantly higher level of interest in teaching the subject in the U.S.A., especially so at medical school level—the teaching of communication skills was already institutionalized in that country, recognized as a legitimate component of the course. Moreover, communication skills training was not only considered appropriate for student doctors. A recent survey by Westberg *et al.* (unpublished) reported that interpersonal skills training figured in no fewer than 30 out of 44 programmes training students to become Physician Assistants.

3 WHAT EFFECT CAN COMMUNICATION SKILLS TRAINING HAVE?

One possible reason why U.K. medical schools do so little in this field could be that there is little or no evidence to suggest that training in communication skills has any significant effect. What is the position? The recent paper by Carroll and Monroe (1979) reviewed 73 studies on the teaching of medical interviewing: the authors conclude that: "instruction in medical interviewing has generally promoted significant gains in students' interview skills as measured by various cognitive tests, affective instruments and observed behaviour". Crucial components of effective teaching included provision for direct observation and feedback on students' interviewing behaviour, structured feedback, and explicit statements of interview skills to be learnt. Another methodological review by Carroll and Monroe (1980) of published reports on communication skills training concludes similarly.

Only limited evaluations have been conducted in the U.K., with the majority taking place in the U.S.A. Studies in Britain have been conducted at Birmingham, Dundee and Oxford. Some of these demonstrated positive change, though one was not evaluated in any strict sense. In the U.S.A. the outcome of training when this has been evaluated has typically resulted in "experimental" trainees functioning at a significantly higher empathy level than their controls.

3.1 An Experimental Evaluation

One of the more carefully controlled experiments in the U.K. to evaluate the effect of an interpersonal skills training programme was that conducted in Cambridge in 1978, described by Pendleton and Wakeford (1979). Here, a group of 22 first year students were randomly assigned to one of two groups, one experimental and the other acting as a control. Students were video-taped at their very first or second patient contact, right at the beginning of the clinical medical course. These video-tapes formed the basis of subsequent training which involved three 60–90 minute tutorials for each student in groups of two or three. These were for the purpose of reviewing the video-tapes and encouraging the students to analyse critically their own performance. The training drew attention to the affective component of doctor/patient inter-action and in particular to the ways in which the patient's feelings can be

Table 13.2. Changes in individuals' scores (max. possible score 200).

	Participant	Before	After	Change
Control Group	1	137	137	0
	2	133	133	0
	3	126	116	−10
	4	144	135	− 9
	5	138	138	0
	6	135	136	+ 1
	7	137	133	
	8	128	137	+ 9
	9	128	136	+ 8
	10	124	122	− 2
Total		1330	1323	
Mean		133	132	
S.D.		6·0	7·0	
Experimental group				
	1	133	143	+10
	2	109	136	+27
	3	114	144	+30
	4	125	141	+16
	5	142	147	+ 5
	6	134	151	+16
	7	118	144	+26
	8	110	140	+30
	9	123	131	+ 8
	10	116	130	+14
	11	124	148	+24
	12	141	152	+11
Total		1489	1707	
Mean		124	142	
S.D.		10·9	7·0	

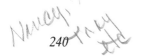

Richard Wakeford

communicated non-verbally.

These training sessions were supplemented by large group meetings of two hours duration. Here again, matters were exemplified with reference to the video-tapes of students in the group.

The control group did not receive such training sessions, but met with the teacher in the normal way throughout the three-week period which was devoted to learning mastery of the basic skills of history taking and the physical examination (so it could be expected that these students also should have improved).

At the end of the three-week period, both groups were video-taped once more, and the video-tapes were then rated by independent raters on a set of pre-determined criteria. The raters were unaware of which students were in control or experimental groups and whether the video-tape was made before or after training (or its absence).

A highly significant improvement took place within the control group, with each member's score improving: no overall change took place within the control group—although some students improved slightly, but others got worse. These results are shown in Table 13.2, and the difference between the groups is highly significant ($P<0.0005$).

Table 13.3 lists the specific skills what the observers were rating and shows significant improvements to have occurred upon each.

Table 13.3. Significance of change of experimental group scores by scale.

	Scale	t score
Specific Skills	Beginning	4.02^a
	Questioning	6.00^b
	Listening	7.30^b
	Regulating	5.05^b
	Coping with the patient's feelings	3.96^a
	Clarifying	5.01^b
Overall Impressions Created by each Participant		
	Warmth	4.75^b
	Confidence	3.97^a
	Involvement	5.81^b
	Effectiveness	5.33^b

[a] $P<0.005$. [b] $P<0.0005$.

Five conclusions were drawn:

(1) Training in communication skills can be carried out effectively in a medical school without a lot of time involvement. It is compatible with the acquisition of basic clinical skills and can be carried out at the commencement of the clinical training of the students.

(2) Training need not consist of modelling the students' behaviour on the competent behaviour of an "expert". Modelling is useful when the student has very little interpersonal competence but it raises problems of congruence when any individual is asked to mimic the behaviour of another individual.

(3) Training can be effective for all students, irrespective of their initial level of interpersonal competence.

(4) Medical students find training in interpersonal skills both useful and enjoyable adjuncts to training in clinical skills.

(5) Evaluation of training needs to be extensive.

4 WHY IS MORE NOT DONE?

Enhancing the effectiveness of doctor–patient communication can improve patient care, and there is ample evidence on both sides of the Atlantic to demonstrate that it is indeed possible to institute effective training in communication skills with relatively little difficulty. Why is it then that so little is done in the U.K.? This chapter concludes with a review of some of the obstacles to change in medical education in this country. Consideration of these will, it is hoped, lead to the possibility of more effective innovation and hence the more general introduction of teaching in communication skills.

Although there is a body of literature on innovation in education generally, there is little which is specific to higher education or medical education in particular.[1] However, a report of the Group for Research and Innovation in Higher Education (1973) describes the conclusions of a group who looked into this problem. Although, as the group point out, nobody has yet revealed a "universal law governing the process of innovation", a number of factors have been identified which can prevent or obstruct innovation and change in higher education in the U.K. First of all, and perhaps most obviously, are the personalities and attitudes of those involved. Frequently, these can be obstructive. However, attitudes—if not personalities—are not immutable. People behave in different ways in different climates of opinion. Thus, the institutional or departmental ethos may have a profound effect on the success or otherwise of an innovation, and indeed upon the attitudes of those concerned.

Past experience of innovation or change has been found to be significant in influencing the success or indeed the occurrence of subsequent innovations.

Poor communication is also important: a frequent reason for innovation failing is that those staff who should have understood the rationale behind it did not do so—this has been found to be particularly important in connection with technical, secretarial and other support staff.

Another difficulty is that innovating programmes often do not have an agreed time span fixed in advance for the innovation to run before it is reviewed. Too often "an attempted change whose results have not lived up to initial expectations (which are in any case usually optimistic) will be taken as providing a valid reason for leaving things as they were before, in spite of the fact that the . . . problems the change was designed to tackle remain stubbornly unresolved". In short, innovations need experimental protection. Finally, dwindling resources will make innovation less likely to occur—unless a clear case can be made for the saving of revenue.

These general observations will almost certainly apply to medical education, but this also has many specific obstacles of its own. There are a number of differences between medical education and the teaching of other university subjects which make its implementation and development particularly difficult. Mostly these stem from matters relating to clinical training, though with increasing integration in medical schools, they are relevant to all sections of most schools' courses. They stem from two principal sources: the complex function of undergraduate medical education, and aspects of the implement-ation of the teaching process itself.

4.1 Some Difficulties of Medical Education

Medicine is a vast subject with a very broad range of knowledge, skills and attitudes that need to be acquired during training for it. Unfortunately, there is much discussion and little agreement between its teachers as to what a student needs to know, or be proficient in by the end of the undergraduate course, with regard to any of its component disciplines. That this is true is known to anyone who has served on a curriculum committee, or who has perhaps tried to persuade a teacher in his medical school to use a tape/slide programme made in another school. This position is compounded by rapid changes both in the theoretical background to medicine and in its practice. Few would disagree with the Harvard Dean who used to say to his new medical students, "Half of what you are taught as medical students will in ten years have been shown to be wrong, and the trouble is, none of your teachers knows which half." Medicine is thus an enormous, growing and changing subject, with—as far as undergraduates' training is concerned—ill-defined boundaries. This makes harsh demands on both the teachers and the students.

These demands are exacerbated if the overall functions of undergraduate medical education are not agreed between the medical school, its teachers and the students. Most of those concerned with organizing this period of training would agree that it has two valid, parallel aims. On the one hand is "education", and on the other "vocational training". The General Medical Council has emphasized the educational aspect in recent years and has urged schools "to ensure that the memorizing and reproduction of factual data should not be allowed to interfere with the primary need for fostering the critical study of principles and the development of independent thought". As Pickering (1956) suggested over 20 years ago, the purpose of the undergraduate course being within a university is "to train the student's mind so that he can collect and verify facts concerning health and disease in man, and so that he can form a balanced judgement on issues that affect both individuals and groups". The vocational requirement of undergraduate medical education is also stated by the GMC:

> By the time of qualification the graduate should have sufficient knowledge of the structure and the functions of the human body in health and disease, of normal and abnormal behaviour, and of the techniques of diagnosis and treatment, to enable him to assume the responsibility of a pre-registration House Officer.

These two aims of the undergraduate period will inevitably conflict, and result in special problems for the medical schools. How, for instance, might a demand from the ENT department for "a fair slice of the curriculum" be reconciled with "the need to foster the critical study of principles"? It is important to recognize that unless medical schools, their teachers and most of all their students are all aware of these two legitimate, parallel aims, such questions will never be answered satisfactorily.

The other principal source of the special problems of medical education in the U.K. is contained within the broad process of its teaching: there are a number of related facets. Possibly the most important of these is the variety of attributes expected in a clinical medical staff member. Most university teachers have responsibility for teaching, research and administration. Over and above the three, clinicians have their clinical responsibilities: not only are these vital to the maintenance of their efficiency as teachers and doctors, but clinical responsibilities must clearly often take priority over other aspects. Clinical school teachers thus tend to be highly able, highly specialized, somewhat unpredictable and very busy. Such factors can often encourage in some teachers an attitude which is not uncommon in higher education generally in the U.K. This attitude denies the difficulties surrounding the teaching/learning process: education is seen as a simple, commonsense affair. Not only is education straightforward, but so are its problems, and these have obvious solutions. Suggestions from educational psychologists and others that matters might possibly be more complicated than they seem and that other explanations are possible, are met with irritation and disbelief.

Another problem in the United Kingdom is that the majority of medical school teachers are not in fact employed by the university. They are consultants and junior clinical staff employed by the National Health Service. Their link with the medical school is tenuous, possibly involving the conferment of some title such as "recognized university teacher", a small amount of money, and occasional communications. The school's level of control over them regarding their teaching of its students is frequently slight, and great variation in student experience therefore results. The position is made even more difficult when the teaching is being carried out in more distant peripheral hospitals, away from the medical school and the teaching hospital: this is an increasingly common practice in the U.K.

4.2 Obstacles to Change Specific to Medical Education

If these are some of the special problems and features of medical education in the U.K., what are the specific obstacles to change to which they (no doubt only in part) lead?

Central control of undergraduate medical education in the U.K. is loose: the G.M.C. does not impose strict time limits for the various components of the medical schools' curricula, for instance, and nor does it indicate in any detail what these components should be. The position is emphasized by the G.M.C.'s guidelines on medical education being called "Recommendations". Whilst, under certain circumstances (in particular, times of growth) loose recommendations may be an effective exhortation to experiment and innovate, in more difficult times they can be used as an excuse for not doing so. Indeed, considering the looseness of the central control, the similarity of the courses in U.K. medical schools is surprising. There is thus no central pressure to introduce teaching on specific, limited topics.

More significant perhaps is the effect of a proposed innovation on a medical school's departments. With the growth of new disciplines such as immunology and new specialities such as oncology, many departments in medical schools have lost teaching time, that frightening traditional indicator of status and importance. Thus, a proposed innovation which takes up teaching time is seen as a threat by the existing departments, who may well together veto such suggestions. This argument applies particularly forcefully to proposed innovations which are non-departmental in origin—just as a communication skills training course might well be.

Many observers would agree that much of the medical profession is characterized by a conservatism in outlook. Whatever its origins, and taken together with the fact that the form and structure of medical education (not its content) is very similar to what it was 30 (or even 60) years ago, this can and does produce the attitude, "What did for me is good enough for you now, my boy". Moreover, since most clinical teachers in medical schools are not paid principally to teach, but to be consultant or junior staff in the National Health Service, they have an apparently legitimate ability to abandon their responsibilities when faced by what they would see as an unacceptable innovation or development. "If you don't like the way I am doing it, then I'll stop doing it altogether".

Surprisingly little work has been done on the professional socialization of medical students, though it has been shown to take place in two reports by Harris (1974) and Coombs (1978). (In this connection, it is interesting to note that in response to what they describe as the "subtle process of dehumanization" of students in the clinical course, Comstock and Williams (1980) have felt the need to introduce in their medical school a "caring skills" course.) The author's experiences in a participant evaluation programme with clinical students over three years have led him to conclude that quite a lot of students mimic certain attitudes of those particular consultants and other staff whom they admire, within weeks of their arrival. This can extend to an accelerated growth of hostile attitudes towards innovations which would alter the *status quo*.

Finally, it must be noted that there is inevitably hostility towards ideas put forward by groups who are identified by the medical profession as undermining its status and questioning its role. Social scientists are the most noteworthy.

5 CONCLUSION

When an attempt is made to introduce the teaching of interpersonal communication skills into an undergraduate medical curriculum—in which one might well regard it as a fundamental component—this is frequently opposed. Many reasons are given, but a common one is "you haven't proved that it will help the medical students". (Of course, few studies have shown that conventional components of medical courses "help the medical students".)

It is through understanding the process of educational innovation the obstacles to it, and the "reward and punishment" characteristics of teaching institutions that more effective and appropriate curricula will be implemented, as opposed to being planned. Between different countries, educational situations vary enormously, however, and this analysis with regard to the U.K. will probably apply only slightly to other countries. Certainly, much additional study of innovation in medical education is needed, but is hoped that this chapter will give the would-be curriculum developer one additional small piece of assistance—though in the case of the introduction of communication skills training it might be thought that the review of 73 research reports quoted above would render this unnecessary. The fact that communication skills training now forms a regular part of the course at Cambridge University School of Clinical Medicine may act as encouragement.

NOTE

1. Since preparation of this chapter, a most readable and interesting paper by Blizard *et al.* (1980) has outlined factors relating to large-scale curriculum change in Indonesian medical schools. His theoretical review is commended to the reader.

REFERENCES

Blizard, P. J., MacMahon, C. M. and Magin, D. J. (1980). Large-scale curriculum change in a system of ten Indonesian medical schools—a case study of educational innovation. *Higher Educ.* **9**, 573–603.
Bryant, G. D. and Norman, G. R. (1979). The communication of uncertainty. In *Proceedings of the 18th Annual Conference on Research in Medical Education.* Washington: American Association of Medical Colleges, pp. 205–207.
Carroll, J. G. and Monroe, J. (1979). Teaching medical interviewing: a critique of educational research and practice. *J. Med. Educ.* **54**, 498–500.
Carroll, J. G. and Monroe, J. (1980). Teaching clinical interviewing in the health professions: a review of empirical research. *Evaluat. Hlth Professions*, **3**, 21–45.
Comstock, L. M. and Williams, R. C. (1980). The way we teach students to care for patients. *Med. Teacher* **2**, 168–170.
Coombs, R. H. (1978). *Mastering Medicine.* The Free Press, New York.
Fletcher, C. (1979). Towards better practice and teaching of communication between doctors and patients. In *Mixed Communications* (G. McLachlan, ed.) pp. 3–41. Nuffield Provincial Hospitals Trust, London.
G.M.C. (1980). *Recommendations as to Basic Medical Education.* General Medical Council, London.
Group for Research and Innovation in Higher Education (1973). *Newsletter*, No. 3. The Nuffield Foundation, London.
Harris, C. M. (1974). Formation of professional attitudes in medical students. *Brit. J. Med. Educ.* **8**, 241–245.
Helfer, R. E. (1970). An objective comparison of the pediatric interviewing skills of freshmen and senior medical students. *Pediatrics* **45**, 623–627.
Junek, W., Burra, P. and Leichner, P. (1979). Teaching interviewing skills by encountering patients. *J. Med. Educ.* **54**, 402–407.
Kahn, G. S., Cohen, B. and Jason, H. (1979). The teaching of interpersonal skills in U.S. medical schools. *J. Med. Educ.* **54**, 29–35.
Pendleton, D. and Wakeford, R. (1979). A communication skills course for new clinical students. Paper presented at the Annual Meeting of the Association for the

Study of Medical Education, University of Southampton, September.

Pickering, G. (1956). The purpose of medical education. *Brit. Med. J.* **ii**, 113–116.

Pickering, G. (1978). Doctor–patient relationship: the impact of recent changes in medicine and society. *Acta Med. Scand.* **204**, 339–343.

Report (1977). *Basic Medical Education in the British Isles: Report of the G.M.C. Survey*. Nuffield Provincial Hospitals Trust, London.

Segall, A. and Roberts, L. W. (1980). A comparative analysis of physician estimates and levels of medical knowledge among patients. *Sociol. Hlth Illness* **2**, 317–334.

Science News (1973). The malpractice crunch: impact on U.S. medicine. **103**, 338–339.

Westberg, J., Kahn, G., Cohen., B. and Friel, T. Teaching interpersonal skills in physician assistant programs: findings of a national survey. (Unpublished paper.)

Working Party (1980) (Chairman, Sir John Walton). *Talking with Patients: a Teaching Approach*. Nuffield Provincial Hospitals Trust, London.

14 The Consultation and Postgraduate General Practice Training

John Hasler

1 HISTORY

Unlike undergraduate medical education, planned postgraduate training is of more recent origin and postgraduate or vocational training for general practice has a very short history indeed. For many years, intending specialists have taken a number of hospital posts to prepare themselves for consultant appointments, but general practitioners have been able to enter practice immediately after the compulsory registration year if they so wished. Until recently many did so, whilst others chose to do one or two more hospital posts before settling. Although at the beginning of the National Health Service it was possible for a young doctor to work for a year in general practice as a trainee, this was largely an apprenticeship and there were complaints of exploitation without much training. By the end of the fifties the number of trainees in general practice was very small compared with today's figures. The first serious attempt to provide some kind of training programme was in Inverness in 1952 when junior hospital appointments were linked to a general practice trainee year. It was not until nearly ten years later that another part of the country—the Wessex region—set up similar appointments with the support of the Nuffield Provincial Hospitals Trust. These were two-year programmes with a traditional obstetrics and gynaecology senior house officer post, a six-month supernumerary hospital post and a traditional trainee year in a local practice. By the second half of the sixties a day-release course was provided for those in the general practice year. Since the early seventies the number of general practice training appointments with day-release courses has expanded rapidly.

Over a decade ago the Royal Commission on Medical Education (1968) adopted the recommendations of the then College of General Practitioners (1966) that a period of vocational training should precede practice as a principal. The length of training was to be five years—two in hospital and three in general practice. For various reasons this has not come about and the current period of training is three years, of which at least one is spent in a training general practice and the remainder in hospital or community medicine posts.

2 EDUCATIONAL AIMS

At the beginning of the seventies, the Royal College of General Practitioners produced an important book (1972) indicating five areas of education relevant for a general practitioner. These were Clinical Practice in Health and Disease, Human Development and Human Relationships, and Society and Medicine, and the Organization of the Practice. This book is still widely used today although the educational aims were revised subsequently by the Second European Conference on the Teaching of General Practice (1974) meeting at Leeuwenhorst in the Netherlands.

The educational aims, however, continue to present problems. Some of these problems are similar to those referred to by Richard Wakeford in his earlier chapter. Not only is medicine a vast subject, but so is general practice. General Practitioners are the only clinicians who do not, by definition, limit their sphere of activities. Although there is overall agreement in broad terms about the scope of general practice, there is much discussion and disagreement about the priorities for vocational training as highlighted by Tate and Pendleton (1980) and Pearce (in preparation). The dilemma between "education" and "vocational training" is another very real one, the majority of general practice trainers and consultants who are after all present primarily to provide a service to patients, believing the most important objective is to get the young doctor to cope as effectively as possible as soon as he can.

3 ORGANIZATION

The responsibility for postgraduate training rests with Regional Postgraduate Committees for Medical Education and their area of responsibility is the same as that of the Regional Health Authority in which they are situated. Each committee is usually made up of representatives of the University and the Health Authorities and each has a Postgraduate Dean who acts as its executive officer. Advice and policy on general practice training comes from a subcommittee for general practice and the day to day general practice responsibility rests with a Regional Adviser for General Practice. Assisting the Regional Adviser there are Associate Regional Advisers and Course Organizers and all these doctors are practising general practitioners for a substantial part of the week.

The two years training in hospital are spent in the main in senior house officer posts of six months' duration in various specialities—commonly obstetrics, gynaecology, paediatrics, general medicine, geriatrics, psychiatry or accident and emergency. These are establishment posts which are adopted by general practice training schemes and included in rotations to make up two hospital years. As with any junior hospital posts, the teaching responsibility rests with the consultant or more often his registrar, most of whom will have had no experience of general practice. The model is different in North America where the hospital training is usually supernumerary to the junior hospital staffing establishment.

The general practice period is spent in a service general practice, specially appointed by the Regional General Practice Subcommittee. Each region sets its own criteria for the practices following national guidelines set by the Joint Committee on Postgraduate Training for General Practice, and certain standards are expected, for example, in records and library facilities. The general practitioner appointed as trainer has to provide some kind of regular tuition and general supervision. General practitioner trainers are paid a trainer's grant in addition to the reimbursement of the trainee's salary. There are a considerable number of courses for trainers to help with the understanding of educational method and many trainers attend regular groups or "workshops".

During the training programme, the trainee will attend a day or half-day release course each week where a variety of topics are presented or discussed, ranging from clinical problems to practice organization and sociological subjects.

Not every trainee will opt for a three year appointment as described above. Some will choose a variety of individual hospital posts and then do twelve months in general practice as a separate appointment.

4 MANDATORY TRAINING

By the end of the seventies the number of trainees had expanded rapidly and by April 1980 there were 2116 in England alone. The number of general practice trainers in England at that time was 1695. An Act of Parliament was passed at the request of the profession to introduce mandatory training before a doctor could practise as a principal in the N.H.S. This means that since February 1981, no one has been able to enter N.H.S. general practice without having done 12 months in a training practice and in August 1982, the other two years became compulsory as well.

5 ASSESSMENT

The Act lays down that training must be done, not that a standard must be reached. Many regions use forms of continuous assessment and a large number of trainees sit the Membership Examination of the Royal College of General Practitioners at the end of their training. This examination consists of written papers and an oral examination and by 1981 more than 1000 doctors a year were taking it.

6 PROBLEMS FACING VOCATIONAL TRAINING

In spite of the rapid explosion in general practice vocational training culminating in the Act of Parliament, many problems remain to be resolved. The two years in hospital are virtually the same for general practice trainees as specialist trainees and may not provide relevant experience throughout. This means that virtually all the learning relating specifically to general practice has to be done in the general practice 12 months, which is too short.

Some of the problems of defining aims and priorities have already been referred to but there are other difficulties mainly related to the fact that the teaching is provided, unlike in North America, by doctors whose main purpose in life is to provide a clinical service to patients. Wakeford in his earlier chapter highlights most of these difficulties and what is true for medical student teachers is also true for those teaching junior hospital doctors and general practice trainees. Thus, clinical responsibilities frequently take priority over teaching, and education is often seen as a simple commonsense affair. Indeed many general practice trainers believe in their heart of hearts that nothing more than an apprenticeship is needed. Central control is difficult to impose and those responsible for general practice training have often to move at the pace of the lowest common denominator. Nevertheless, in spite of all these difficulties, we have found that it is possible to get general practice trainers in the Oxford region to monitor consultations and to learn the appropriate skills.

7 COMMUNICATION SKILLS

7.1 The Need

Medical undergraduate training takes place largely in hospital. All medical schools now have some contribution from doctors who work outside the hospital, such as general practitioners and epidemiologists, but the contribution is small in proportion to the whole curriculum.

The fact that most of the undergraduate medical experience is in hospital means that many problems are relatively acute and primarily seen as physical as opposed to a mix of physical, psychological and social. Furthermore, patients have to a large extent been sorted and classified by the time they reach hospital. Medical students tend to acquire a limited style of questioning and history taking appropriate to how they perceive these problems.

This may be one reason why medical school teachers, with the exception of psychiatrists and general practitioners, tend to be far more interested in the development of technical knowledge and skills than in social skills such as communication between doctor and patient, quite apart from the more general difficulties previously described. Wakeford (Chapter 13, this volume), describes a method of helping medical students to understand communication skills. There is little evidence, however, that many medical schools are attempting this, and Wakeford shows that in 1975–1977 approximately one third of British medical schools offered no training at all in this field.

Unless he has been to a medical school where communication skills are taught, the young doctor on qualification is unaware of a whole facet of dealing with patients. His hospital background from medical school is now reinforced by 12 months as a pre-registration house officer where he will deal again with the admission and management of a large number of patients with acute medical and surgical conditions. He will be busy, unsure and supervised by doctors possessing skills and interests in technical medicine. It is this doctor, who may at the end of the year, decide to enter a general practice training scheme.

As we have seen, two out of three years are now spent in more hospital posts reinforcing the previous experience. Unless the trainee works, during the two years, in a psychiatry department, where communication skills are taught, or has had training in this field as a medical student, he arrives at his general practice year unaware of the skills he will need. Whether he achieves these skills in the training practice largely depends on the interest and knowledge of the local course organizer or general practice trainer at the present time.

What we would ultimately like to see is the teaching of communication skills in both undergraduate and post-graduate phases of training. As far as general practice is concerned at present, we have to assume that doctors have had no specific training. But even if communication skills do become taught widely at undergraduate level, there will always be a need for specific training for the consultation in general practice.

It is here for the first time the doctor comes to grips with patients with undifferentiated symptoms. The woman with a headache may have sinusitis, temporal arteritis, herpes zoster, or much more likely anxiety. The young trainee finds difficulty in disentangling the emotional from the physical. Added to this he is lacking in confidence.

We have found that trainees' difficulties in the main are largely predictable. They tend to use closed rather than open questions since it is the former that have been learnt in hospital and are appropriate there. For the same reason reflected questions do not appear much in the trainee's vocabulary. He or she finds using silence difficult, particularly when anxious or unsure. The straightforward physical problems are relatively easy but patients with ill-defined or emotional difficulties and those used to manipulating the doctor cause great problems. After approximately eight years almost entirely spent in hospital our young doctor finds that the style and skills he has used are often inappropriate and he has to go back to square one.

Much of general practice is spent in dealing with patients with psychological problems or in situations where it is not clear what the problem is. Closed questions often confuse the issue further and may hinder the identification of the problem. Alternatively, the young doctor may have some idea of how to word the questions but fails to convey his real interest by inappropriate non-verbal behaviour. Trainees have often been taught as medical students that the doctor's role is unimportant or passive, and this may be interpreted as uninterest by the patient.

Much of general practice is spent trying to persuade people to change their behaviour or life style and these aspects have been referred to in earlier chapters. Some doctors consider that all consultations should have a health education component. But if general practitioners are unaware of what style and techniques are appropriate, how will they make the most impact?

Without specific help, the young doctor may eventually discover some of the techniques for himself but in many cases may adopt a standard style which is frequently inappropriate.

7.2 Organization of Teaching

The essential factor in any teaching and learning of communication skills between doctor and patient is to be able to witness and analyse real life consultations and general practice is no exception. Audiovisual teaching material can demonstrate consultations and certain techniques taken from real life, but ultimately the doctor must be able to analyse and improve his own performance.

The first step in a training practice is for the general practitioner trainer and trainee to agree at the beginning of the trainee's attachment that analysis of the trainee's consultations will be essential. We have found that the establishment of ground rules at the start of the trainee attachment is much more likely to succeed than if one tries to change matters half way through. This is particularly true of consultation analysis because trainees feel anxious at being watched and are more likely to accept it if it is part of the programme from the first week. Reluctance by the trainee is not just due to anxiety at being monitored. Examining consultations may make matters temporarily more clumsy and just at the time when young doctors are trying to establish their clinical independence, the very basis on which they practise medicine is being questioned and adjusted.

We have found it useful to establish a certain method of proceeding, and Schofield enlarges on this in his chapter. Briefly, we start with the analysis of video-recorded consultations of other doctors to allow familiarity with the technique. It is important that any analysis starts with identifying strengths first and only subsequently identifying weaknesses. Then we suggest that the trainee observes or monitors his trainer's consultations and finally allows himself to be observed.

How the monitoring takes place is a matter for the two people concerned. The way most commonly adopted in the United Kingdom is for the second doctor to sit in the consulting room. It is easy and sometimes appears to be ethically more acceptable but it suffers from two disadvantages. One is that the presence of a third party, particularly if well known to the patient, can distort the consultation and secondly there is no means of playing the consultation back so that the trainee can see and hear himself.

In 1980 3127 questionnaires were distributed to trainees in the United Kingdom for data which were presented to the Fourth National Trainee Conference at Exeter and analysed in a Royal College of General Practitioners Occasional Paper (1981). Only 29% of trainees in their general practice year reported that their trainer regularly sat in on them, although this figure hides a wide variation from 68% in one region to 4% in another.

Probably the second most common method in use today in the U.K. is audiotape. It is relatively simple and cheap and can be played back afterwards. Much of the stimulation for this type of analysis came from the work by Byrne and Long (1976) in the Department of General Practice in Manchester. They showed how it is possible to break down the phases of the consultation and drew attention to the tendency for the general practitioner to adopt a standard style regardless of the kind of patient and problem being dealt with. Audiotape does not demonstrate the non-verbal behaviour of the doctor and patient, but nevertheless it should be standard equipment now for every training practice. Only 16% of trainees from the 1980 Exeter Survey reported regular taped consultations with a range of 35%–0%.

One of the least used methods to date in the U.K. is the two-way mirror. This is in contrast to North America where many family medicine residents are monitored frequently through mirrors. It is surprising that so few practices have installed what is after all a relatively inexpensive facility. Trainees working in practices, where two-way mirrors are in use, say they prefer it to having another doctor in the room. Milligan and Stewart (1981) found that the majority of patients had no objection.

However, undoubtedly the ideal method is videotape recording allowing trainer and trainee, and a larger audience if desired, to watch the consultation together and stop it where they will. Until recently it seemed unlikely that individual training practices would be able to achieve this, but in the Oxford region in 1979, following increasing interest by trainers and trainees, a portable video-recording deck, camera and monitor were purchased for use on courses and in practices. By 1981 all schemes had video-recording equipment available for all their training practices and a number of practices had their own equipment installed permanently.

7.3 Difficulties

In Britain, in spite of the comments referred to previously in relation to the Oxford region, it should not be thought that consultation analysis for general practice trainees is widespread or generally accepted yet. Many trainers still believe that communicating with patients comes naturally to all doctors. This is largely because their own training has been deficient and because they have not been taught the techniques of doing it. Unless a trainer has learnt these techniques or is unusually perceptive he will concentrate on clinical aspects of the consultation, such as whether a physical examination was made appropriately, or if the right antibiotic was prescribed and so on. It is necessary therefore to provide courses for trainers where the skills may be learnt, and one such course is now provided regularly in the Oxford Region. Until they have learnt the necessary techniques, the trainer and trainee will invent various reasons why the exercise is a waste of time.

In parts of North America matters seem to have gone almost to the other extreme and trainees (residents) and medical students are observed frequently either on video or by two-way mirror. In Australia the frequency of monitoring seems to be roughly the same as in Britain.

8 CONCLUSION

Although communication skill-learning has been frequently non-existent in

Britain, there are signs now that things are changing. There is still a great need for trainers to learn consultation analysis skills. It is to be hoped that in the next few years the majority of trainees will have their consultations regularly observed and analysed.

REFERENCES

Byrne, P. S. and Long, B. E. L. (1976). *Doctors Talking to Patients.* H.M.S.O., London.

College of General Practitioners (1966). Evidence of the College to the Royal Commission on Medical Education. *Reports from General Practice No. 5.* R.C.G.P., London.

Fourth National Trainee Conference, Exeter 1980 (1981). Occasional Paper 18, Royal College of General Practitioners.

Milligan, J. M. and Stewart, T. I. (1981). The Two-Way Mirror. *Trainee*, Update Publications, 1.3. 116–118.

Pearce, J. (in preparation).

Royal College of General Practitioners (1972). *The Future General Practitioner: Learning and Teaching.* B.M.A., London.

Royal Commission on Medical Education (1968). *Report 1965–68.* H.M.S.O., London.

Second European Conference on the Teaching of General Practice (1974). The General Practitioner in Europe. Statement by the Working Party, Leeuwenhorst, Netherlands.

Tate, P. H. L. and Pendleton, D. A. (1980). Why not tear up the European Aims? *J. Roy. Coll. Gen. Pract.* **30**, 743.

15 The Application of the Study of Communication Skills to Training for General Practice

Theo Schofield

1 INTRODUCTION

It was in 1960 that Sir James Spence wrote that "The essential unit of medical practice is . . . a consultation, and all else in the practice of medicine derives from it". In 1972 it was stated in "The Future General Practitioner—Learning and Teaching", a book reviewing the knowledge skills and attitudes that were essential for general practice, that "The consultation is central to the whole of this report".

It is, however, only very recently that many of the vocational training schemes for general practice in the United Kingdom have started to include training in communication skills in the curriculum. Hasler (1978) reviewed reports by trainees in teaching practices in the Oxford Region, and found that 24 out of 54 trainees had not received any joint consultations or monitoring sessions throughout their year as a trainee, and there is every reason to believe that the same was true in the majority of the other regions in the United Kingdom.

In his chapter in this volume, Hasler has reviewed the organization of Vocational Training for General Practice and described the recent introduction of communication skills training in the Oxford Region. In this chapter I will be describing some of the difficulties that we have encountered and our approach in overcoming them.

2 RECOGNIZING OUR DEFICIENCIES

Byrne and Long (1976) in their major study of 2500 general practitioner consultations described a remarkable lack of variation in style by individual doctors and concluded that some styles were quite inadequate for dealing with non-organic illnesses. This report and the work of the Department of General Practice at Manchester has been very influential in highlighting the deficiencies in our current practice, and by implication the failure of our current methods of training.

Marks *et al.* (1979) described the variation between General Practitioners in their ability to detect psychiatric illness in their patients. On average only 54% of mood disorders that were predicted to be present by a psychiatric screening questionnaire were recognized by the doctor.

Other studies have looked at the outcome of consultations, particularly using the measures of information gathering by the doctor, information transfer to the patient, patient compliance and patient satisfaction. Many of these studies have revealed outcomes which are much less than optimal and some are described and discussed by Pendleton, Ley and Cartwright in their chapters in this volume (Chapters 1, 4 and 9).

One of the reasons that these deficiencies can go unrecognized is that none of these outcomes can be determined by the doctor alone without reference to the patients, either from their statements and behaviour within the consultation, or by subsequent enquiry. If as doctors we fail to have this awareness, it is quite possible to continue to believe that we have defined fully our patients problems, that the explanations that we have given have been understood, that the patients are following our treatment and are satisfied with the care that they have received.

3 COLLABORATION WITH OTHER DISCIPLINES

There is a tendency for doctors to believe that the consultations between doctors and patients are unique, and that because they appear to be able to perform the task they are also able to teach others to do so. It is, however, one of many types of interview between a caring professional and a patient or client, and we have much to learn from disciplines such as social psychology and sociology, which have studied the content and context of these interviews, and also from other professionals who have therapeutic relationships with their clients.

Most vocational training schemes in this country have had little contact with members of these disciplines, though the situation is very different in residency programs in the United States. Hornsby and Kerr (1979) found that

90% of residency programs had at least one faculty member teaching behavioural science. Fifty-four per cent of these were non-physicians while of the physicians 46% were psychiatrists.

The commonest topics that were taught were interviewing skills and interpersonal communication skills. Kahn (1979) found that 88% of Family Practice residency programs included formal training in communication skills and that 88% of these programs used video-technology for teaching, monitoring and feedback.

The Department of General Practice in Manchester which has been so influential in drawing general practitioner teachers' attention to doctors' deficiencies in consultations, has also been a pioneer in developing collaboration with behavioural scientists in general practitioner teaching. The developments of communication skill training in the Oxford Region have been entirely due to our close collaboration with a Social Psychologist, and a variety of studies have come out of this mutually beneficial collaboration.

4 DECIDING WHAT TO TEACH

The only justification for teaching a particular communication skill is the effectiveness of that skill in achieving a particular task in the consultation. It is therefore, necessary to define what it is that we wish to achieve in a consultation. This is difficult.

Individual doctors have widely varying beliefs about their role, and Balint in his book "The Doctor, his Patient and the Illness" (1957) described these beliefs as the doctors "Apostolic Function". He emphasized the need for general practitioners to be able to make "a deeper diagnosis" and develop a more comprehensive understanding of the patient's concerns and behaviour. Browne and Freeling (1976) also described the special function of the general practitioner as "to understand the whole of his patient's communication" so that he could assess the whole person and be able to consider the effect of any intervention in an illness upon the whole life of his patient.

Other writers have taken a different view of the potential of the primary care consultation.

Stott and Davis (1979) proposed a four point framework which had been found to be helpful for general practitioners who try to achieve greater "breadth" in each consultation.

The four points were: (a) management of presenting problems; (b) modification of help seeking behaviour; (c) management of continuing problems; (d) opportunistic health promotion.

Patients also have a wide variety of aims and expectations when consulting their doctor.

It is therefore essential for the definition of tasks for a consultation to be broad and flexible enough to encompass variations in both doctors and patients. This has been described as attempting to provide a "bespoke rather than an off-the-peg consultation".

The approach that we have adopted is to define the tasks for the doctor in terms of meeting the needs of patients. These then include discovering the reasons for the patient's attendance and their ideas, concerns and expectations, sharing understanding with the patient, and involving the patient in their own management. This is a patient-centred approach (see below) and has been expressed in a Consultation Task Rating Scale (Pendleton *et al.*, in press).

The other reason for defining these as the tasks for the consultation is their relationship to desired outcomes. David Pendleton in Chapter 1 has described the sequence of outcomes as immediate, intermediate and long-term. Immediate outcomes include patient satisfaction with the consultation, his memory for and understanding of the doctor's explanations and instructions, and changes in the patient's concern about his problem. Intermediate outcomes include patient compliance with the management, and the long-term outcomes that are desired are changes in the health status and health understanding of the patient.

In Chapter 1 he has reviewed the evidence that links the tasks to be performed within the consultation, or its process, with these outcomes, and has demonstrated that the achievement of the long-term outcomes is dependent on the achievement of the shorter-term outcomes.

The desired doctor–patient relationship has been defined in terms of helping to achieve these tasks rather than in terms of any value judgement of good or bad. The tasks are:

(1) To define the reasons for the patients attendance in physical, psychological and social terms: (a) nature and history of problems; (b) aetiology; (c) patient's ideas, concerns and expectations; (d) effects of problems.

(2) To consider other problems: (a) continuing problems; (b) at risk factors.

(3) To choose an appropriate action for each problem.

(4) To achieve a shared understanding of the problems with the patient.

(5) To involve the patient in the management and encourage him to accept appropriate responsibility.

(6) To use time and resources appropriately: (a) in the consultation; (b) long-term.

(7) To establish or maintain a relationship with the patient which helps to achieve the other tasks.

Freeman *et al.* (1972) showed that the outcome of the medical consultations as measured in terms of patient satisfaction and compliance were found to be favourably influenced by having a physician who is friendly, expressed solidarity, took time to discuss non-medical subjects, and gave the impression of offering information freely.

Balint (1957) took a similar but longer-term view of the dynamics of the doctor–patient relationship, describing it as a "mutual investment company" with the general practitioner gradually acquiring valuable capital invested in his patient, and, vice versa, the patient acquiring a very valuable capital bestowed in his general practitioner. This capital could then be used to yield returns to doctor and patient.

It is now possible for the teacher and learner to consider the skills that are most effective at achieving these tasks. This can be done either by the teacher referring to published work, such as that of Argyle or Ley, a didactic approach, or by the learner observing or testing different methods, a discovery method.

One difficulty with this latter approach is that the degree of achievement of some of these tasks is difficult to determine and all are impossible without reference to the patient. This difficulty applies equally to the doctor and to the observers of the consultation, but can be overcome by some of the methods to be described.

5 SKILLS AND ATTITUDES

Balint in "The Doctor, his Patient and the Illness" (1957) explored the reasons for doctor's difficulties in examining psychological problems in consultations. One factor was lack of skill. He felt the major factor, however, was doctors avoiding personal involvement and the need for self-examination when talking to patients with problems that were often shared by the doctor.

The training methods that he pioneered were based on weekly group case discussions. Their aim was to help doctors become more sensitive to what was going on, consciously or unconsciously, when doctor and patient were together. This approach has great strengths. It allows members of a group not only to acquire new skills but also to discover the discrepancies between their actual behaviour and their intentions and beliefs. This is not a comfortable process but with skilful leadership and with group support it can be accomplished. Balint concluded that the acquisition of new psycho-thera-peutic skills did not consist only of learning something new: it inevitably entailed a limited, though considerable change in the doctor's personality.

This approach does, however, have one major limitation. The group can only directly observe behaviours within the group, and while there will be marked similarities, it is not a complete analogue of the doctor's behaviours and skills in the consultation. Engel (1971) discussed the deficiencies of the case presentation as a method of clinical teaching and makes the point that direct observation is required to determine students' interviewing skills.

Byrne in his earlier study with Long (1976) used audiotape to record interviews, but more recently emphasized the importance of including visual non-verbal behaviour in observations in a study with Heath (1980).

Marks *et al.* (1979) also found that the doctor's personality rather than his interviewing style was the major determinant of his ability to detect psychiatric illness in his patients, though there were interactions between these two factors, and they concluded that attention should also be paid to teaching general practitioners specific interviewing skills.

While it is true that there are attitudes that either facilitate or hinder the doctor from using these skills, it is also true in our experience that the acquisition of new skills and experiencing their effectiveness can alter these attitudes.

6 COURSES FOR TRAINERS AND TRAINEES

There are now many studies evaluating methods of teaching of interviewing skills to medical students such as those described by Jason (1971), Werner and Schneider (1974), Rutter and Maguire (1976), Maguire *et al.* (1978), and Richard Wakeford in this volume. There are others relating to established general practitioners including those of Bird and Lindley (1979), and Verby *et al.* (1979). There are numerous reports of effective teaching methods in American Family Practice residency programs, and a recent report by Davis *et al.* (1980) describing the application of these techniques to General Practice trainees in Cardiff.

Pendleton *et al.* (1978) have previously described the outline of the collaborative research and training programmes which is being developed in the Oxford Region. The initial phases began with two interview studies to help identify communication difficulties both for patients and doctors, and the development of the Consultation Tasks Rating Scale already described. In addition a behavioural description category scheme has been developed so that we can attempt to judge which behaviours are more or less effective at achieving particular tasks.

The next stage has been to teach trainers to use this method of analysis and to apply it to teaching their trainees. This training has been included in the last three annual five-day residential courses for general practitioner teachers described by Schofield and Havelock (in press).

The reason for concentrating first on the trainers was that the opportunity and resources for teaching trainees directly were limited. The trainees attend a three-day residential course early in their year in general practice, and an introduction to communication skills training has been included in this course. They subsequently attend regular small group discussions in their districts, but receive the bulk of their teaching and their experience in their own practices. It was also considered important for the trainees to be able to relate their teaching to their experience in practice. This model of making faculty or teacher training an integral part of the course has also been described by Werner and Schneider (1974).

The design of the first part of the residential courses both for teachers and for trainees is similar. First there is a factual presentation of the concepts of communication skill training, followed by a discussion of pre-recorded consultations selected to exemplify teaching points. The members of the course are asked to explore the tasks in the consultation and the skills required to achieve them. In the early courses the Task Rating Scales and behavioural description scheme were introduced in this first session.

This method of starting by presenting a model for the consultation is essentially similar to many other courses described in the literature, though there is considerable variation in the methods used to develop the model as exemplified by Werner and Schneider (1974), Rutter and Maguire (1976) and Cassata *et al.* (1979).

Maguire *et al.* (1977) compared the history taking skills of three groups of students who had received different courses in communication skills. The first group received two seminars, each of which started with the distribution of printed handouts, the first describing the questions to be asked when taking a history, the second how to interview. This was then followed in each session by discussion of video-taped material. The second group discussed the same material but were asked to suggest themselves which questions should be asked and how to conduct an interview. The same handouts were only given to them at the end of the seminars. The third group of students received a traditional didactic course on communication skills without the use of handouts or video-taped material. The first two courses were both shown to be more effective than the traditional course and there was a clear tendency for the students who used the discovery-mode to obtain better results than those who received the more didactic course.

Our impression, though we have not tested it experimentally, is that our teaching has been more effective, and certainly more acceptable, on those courses in which the members have explored for themselves which skills appear to be more or less effective, than on the earlier courses when they were presented with what could be easily perceived as a "model consultation".

The next phase of the courses for trainers and those for trainees is similar in structure though the purpose is quite different. During this phase the members of the course work in small groups and witness one of their members interviewing a simulated patient in front of the group. The purpose of this exercise for the trainers is to allow them to learn to analyse a consultation and to give feedback to the doctor consulting. It also allows them to explore within the group the difficulties and discomforts of giving and receiving criticism.

The purpose of these discussions for the trainees is for them to begin to explore the use of different communication skills and to receive feedback on their own skills. It also gives them the opportunity to learn to work in a small group.

The simulated patients have been psychology students or members of an amateur dramatic society who have been provided with a "brief" describing the patient and the situation that they are being asked to portray. This method, which has also been described by Jason *et al.* (1971) and Meadow and Hewitt (1972), offers considerable advantages. The simulated patient can provide a fairly constant portrayal of a problem which can be chosen to suit the level and purposes of the course. It is also possible for a learner to interview the patient again exploring the use of different skills after he has received feedback on his first interview, and this can be a very valuable learning experience. Care must be exercised, however, in allowing different doctors in the group to interview the same patient as comparisons between individuals can easily become invidious.

The greatest advantage of using simulated patients is that they are available to participate in the discussion and provide feedback after the interview. I have already discussed the difficulty in assessing the degree of achievement of patient-centred goals without reference to the patient, and the patient's reactions and response to the interview can be very different to those of other observers.

Small groups are used both for economy of time and resources, and for their educational advantages. Verby *et al.* (1979) have described a course which was effective at improving the interviewing skills of a group of experienced general practitioners who met regularly to discuss video-taped recordings of their own consultations. This method of peer review can be widely applied.

7 RULES FOR EFFECTIVE AND ACCEPTABLE FEEDBACK

Giving feedback to a doctor after his consultation has been observed either by an individual teacher or a group is a skilful task. A teacher needs to be able to analyse the skills used in a consultation, identify those that are more or less effective, and be able to reach more effective skills. Due to our lack of training and contact with other disciplines, the majority of trainers do not possess these skills, and are limited therefore, to making value judgements, often using the only available criterion, comparison with their own style.

Using the same argument that has already been applied to communication skills themselves, it follows that some methods of giving feedback are more effective than others, and that these can be learned.

Feedback is more effective if it focuses on specific behaviours and events in the consultation, such as an interruption by the doctor, rather than if it consists of more general statements such as "you never allow the patient to talk". Feedback should be limited to behaviours that can be modified rather than comments on personality such as "you are domineering" which implies a more fixed behaviour pattern. It is also valuable to limit the number of comments to those that can be used by the learner, and to avoid the temptation to overload them with every observation that we are able to make.

One method that has been described by Kagan (1969) and used by Werner and Schneider in their course (1974) is Interpersonal Process Recall. The learner is recorded on video-tape conducting an interview, and the recording is then reviewed by the learner and the teacher together. It is the learner, however, who selects the aspects of the interview that he wishes to be discussed, and the teacher's efforts are devoted to helping the student to describe and understand what he experienced and what he did, rather than to justify or defend his behaviour. They have shown that this is an effective self-learning model.

Ross and Johnson (unpublished data) have described the methods which have been developed in the Department of Family Medicine in the Medical University of South Carolina. After an introductory course which included training in communication skills, each resident was observed and his strengths and weaknesses were evaluated. This information was shared with the resident, and goals for his education in this area over the next six months were mutually agreed. At regular intervals the residents were observed while interviewing patients in the clinic, and the subsequent discussions with a behavioural scientist were directed towards the goals agreed by the resident. The progress of the resident towards achieving these goals is reviewed every six months and this gave the opportunity of evaluating the feedback that had been given.

The principle underlying both these methods is that teaching is more effective if it is directed towards the learner's own goals. Teaching should aim to help the learner develop skills that are effective at achieving chosen outcomes. It is for the learner to decide the outcomes that he wishes to achieve.

There is a widespread feeling that the ways in which a doctor deals with his patients are expressions of his personality. This is particularly true if the doctor has developed his own consultation style without any training during his medical career. The individual behaviours that we acknowledge in ourselves are more likely to be pleasant than those that we choose to ignore. Having these unacknowledged behaviours brought to our attention is therefore uncomfortable. If, in addition, our behaviours are criticized then this discomfort will be increased, and if we have caused discomfort by our criticisms we will also become uncomfortable.

Both these discomforts can interfere with the giving and receiving of effective feedback.

We have attempted to reduce this difficulty, as well as meeting the need to provide feedback that concentrates on developing effective skills and is directed towards the learner's own goals by formulating three rules for commenting on consultations described by Pendleton *et al.* (in press).

These are:

(1) After the consultation has been observed the doctor concerned should be allowed to make the first comments about the consultation and his strengths and weaknesses.

(2) The teacher should first comment on the strengths of the consultation, the tasks that have been achieved and the skills and strategies that were effective in doing so.

(3) Negative comments about tasks which have been less well achieved should always be coupled with constructive comment about skills and strategies that may be more helpful or effective.

Our experience and evaluation of our courses has shown that this approach is effective at assisting learners to become more aware of the skills that they possess that are effective, and to acquire new and more effective skills. The use of these tasks has encouraged learners to be more aware of the importance and effectiveness of using the patient's own ideas, concerns and expectations in the consultation. We also believe that our avoidance of using a prescribed set of skills and our insistence on the rules for giving feedback has contributed considerably to the acceptability of this approach both to trainers and trainees.

8 ETHICAL ISSUES

Two concerns in this area have been expressed. The first is that recording consultations invades the privacy of the doctor–patient relationship and could distort the doctor's and the patient's behaviour. The second is a concern for the confidentiality of the recordings both for the patient and for the doctor.

Our experience has been similar to that of Byrne and Long (1976) and Verby *et al.* (1979), that the recording of consultations is acceptable to the large majority of patients. They are asked beforehand to consent to the consultation being recorded, and asked afterwards whether they wish the recording to be erased, or to give written permission for the tape to be kept and be shown to other doctors.

It is remarkable how little apparent disturbance the camera causes to the process of the consultation, and doctors have reported that they find the presence of a camera in the room far less disturbing than that of another doctor.

Care must be taken in the selection and the use of these recordings in teaching sessions to protect the doctor from unjustified adverse criticism, particularly if he is not present at the discussion.

9 PROVISION OF TIME AND RESOURCES

Apart from the other issues already discussed the other major factors that limit the development of communication skills training are lack of time and of equipment.

Reviewing and discussing recorded consultations is very time consuming but it is our experience that as the value of this training is increasingly recognized, time is found, both in the training groups, and in the practices, for this training to take place.

Hasler (Chapter 14) has described the rapid increase in the availability of portable video-recording equipment in the Oxford Region, so that it is now possible for all trainees to be recorded while consulting in their own practices. It is our aim that this will be used so that every trainee will continue to receive training in communication skills throughout their time in practice.

10 CONCLUSIONS

There is evidence that many general practitioners need to develop their consulting skills, and a strong case for including communication skill training in the curriculum for doctors entering general practice. Training methods have been developed by other behavioural science disciplines, and their application in general practice is greatly assisted by collaboration with these disciplines.

I have described the approach that has been adopted in the Oxford Region Vocational Training Schemes. We have distinguished between the tasks of a consultation and the skills that enable them to be achieved. The tasks have been chosen in the light of a broad, patient-orientated, approach to patient care, and of the evidence linking the process of the consultation to desired outcomes.

The teaching methods described have been used to assist learners to develop skills that are effective at achieving their own aims, and to make the teaching acceptable to both learner and teacher. The availability of portable video-recording equipment has made it possible for these methods to be applied in general practice.

REFERENCES

Balint (1957). *The Doctor, His Patient and the Illness.* Pitman, London.

Bird, J. and Lindley, P. (1979) Interviewing skill: the effects of ultra-brief training for general practitioners. A preliminary report. *Med. Educ.* **13**, 349–355.

Browne, K. and Freeling (1976). *The Doctor–Patient Relationship,* 2nd ed. Churchill Livingstone, London and Edinburgh.

Byrne, P. S. and Heath, C. C. (1980). Practitioners' use of nonverbal behaviour in real consultations. *J. Roy. Coll. Gen. Pract.* **30**, 327–331.

Byrne, P. S. and Long, B. E. (1976). *Doctors Talking to Patients.* H.M.S.O., London.

Cassata, Dm., Conroe, R. M. and Clements, P. W. (1977). A program for enhancing medical interviewing using video-tape feedback in the family practice residency. *J. Family Pract.* **4**, 673–677.

Davis, R. H., Jenkins, M, Smail, S. A. *et al.* (1980). Teaching with audiovisual recordings of consultations. *J. Roy. Coll. Gen. Pract.* **30**, 333–335.

Engel, G. L. (1971). The deficiencies of the case presentation as a method of clinical teaching. *New Eng. J. Med.* **284**, 20–24.

Freeman, B, Negrete, V. F., Davis, M. and Korsch, B. M. (1971). Gaps in doctor–patient communication: doctor–patient interaction analysis. *Pediat. Res.* **5**, 298–311.

Hasler, J. C. (1978). Training practices in the Oxford Region. *J. Roy. Coll. Gen. Pract.* **23**, 353–354.

Hornsby, J. L. and Kerr, R. M. (1979). Behavioural science and family practice: a status report. *J. Family Pract.* **8**, 299–304.

Jason, H., Kagan, N., Werner Am *et al.* (1971). New approaches to teaching basic interview skills to medical students. *Am. J. Psychiat.* **127**, 140–143.

Kagan, N., Schauble, P., Resnikoff, A. *et al.* (1969). Interpersonal recall, *J. Nerv. Ment. Dis.* **148**, 365–374.

Kahn, G., Cohen, B. and Jason, H. (1979). Teaching interpersonal skills in family practice, results of a national survey. *J. Family Pract.* **8**, 309–316.

Maguire, G. P., Clarke, D. and Jolley, B. (1977). An experimental comparison of three courses in history-taking skills for medical students. *Med. Educ.* **11**, 175–182.

Maguire, P., Roe, P., Goldberg, D. *et al.* (1978). The value of feedback in teaching interviewing skills to medical students. *Psycholog. Med.* **8**, 695–704.

Marks, J. N., Goldberg, D. P. and Hillier, V. F. (1979). Determinants of the ability of general practitioners to detect psychiatric illness. *Psycholog. Med.* **9**, 337–353.

Meadow, R. and Hewitt, C. (1972). Teaching communication skills with the help of actresses and video-tape simulation. *Br. J. Med. Educ.* **6**, 317–322.

Pendleton, D., Schofield, T. and Furnham, A. (1978). Social psychology in medical practice and training. *Bull Br. Psychol. Soc.* **31**, 386–387.

Pendleton, D., Schofield, T., Tate, P. and Havelock, P. (in press). *The Consultation, an Approach to Learning and Teaching.* Oxford University Press, Oxford.

Royal College of General Practitioners (1972). The Future General Practitioners. Learning and Teaching, London. *Br. Med. J.*

Rutter, D. R. and Maguire, G. P. (1976). History-taking for medical students II: Evaluation of a Training Programme. *The Lancet* 558–560.

Spence, J. (1960). The need for understanding to individual as part of the training and function of doctors and nurses. *The Purpose and Practice of Medicine.* Oxford University Press, Oxford.

Stott, N. C. H. and Davis, R. H. (1979). The exceptional potential in each primary care consultation. *J. Roy. Coll. Gen. Pract.* **29**, 201–205.

Verby, J. E., Holden, P. and Davis, R. H. (1979). Peer review of consultations in primary care: the use of audiovisual recordings. *Br. Med. J.* 1686–1688.

Werner, A. and Schneider, J. M. (1974). Teaching Medical Students Interactional Skills, A Research-Based Course in the Doctor–Patient Relationship. *New Eng. J. Med.* **290**, 1232–1237.

Part V
Conclusion

16   *Communication in General Practice: New Consultations for Old*

Marshall Marinker

1 INTRODUCTION

The previous chapters suggest that teaching about the consultation has become an unremarkable part of medical school education and of vocational training for general practice. More recently an analysis of the consultation has been recommended in general practice performance review. At the same time consultation research has become a burgeoning field, especially for those behavioural scientists concerned with medicine. How has this come about? What are our intentions, and what is the direction in which we are likely to move? What will be the partnership between doctors and behavioural scientists in these endeavours? What will be the effect on the practice of medicine and the care of patients?

2 HOW HAS THIS COME ABOUT?

Traditionally the consultation, classically the bedside consultation, provided a setting for clinical teaching. The patient was presented as a puzzle, and the intention of the consultation was simply to unravel the mystery. The more arcane the puzzle, the more confounding or well-hidden the clues, the greater the need for skill on the part of the investigator. Those elements in the transaction which had to do with humane behaviour—for example courtesy, gentleness in handling the patient's body, delicacy of feeling in the way in which the body was allowed to be draped at different phases of the physical examination—were displayed as bedside manner. It became part of the folk

humour of modern medical education that clinical eminence often went hand
in hand with a certain brusqueness of manner.

An interest in teaching about the consultation has paralleled the growing
interest in ambulatory care as a setting for medical school education. It may be
that general practice was first introduced into the medical school because it was
thought to be socially relevant, or even educationally trendy. But in the past
few years there has been a growing awareness that the clinical puzzles to be
solved in the general practitioner's consulting room are of a different order
from those presented in the hospital bed and not simply the same puzzles
presented at an earlier or later point in their natural history. Central to the
research of departments of general practice has been the application of
epidemiological methods, occasionally to the study of natural history, but
much more commonly to health services research. Central to the teaching of
general practice has been the consultation. The literature suggests that this
teaching has in some way tried to reconcile a traditionally based problem-
solving approach, a sociologically based exploration of roles, and something
else, something special to general practice which we hint at, rarely describe
and shrink from examining.

3 WHAT ARE OUR INTENTIONS?

Kuhn (1962) distinguishes a revolutionary phase of scientific development
from what he calls "normal science". The terms "revolutionary" and
"normal" refer not to any particular quality of the work which is being done,
nor to its originality. It refers rather to the field of beliefs and practices in which
the work is conceived, and with which it is concerned.

For example, research on the communications between doctor and patient
takes place within that field of scientific endeavour where an analysis of verbal
and non-verbal behaviours is normative: where such measurements are
expected and are to be valued as descriptions and predictions of other human
encounters. It will have a comfortable relationship on the one hand with the
ethological study of primates, and with the study of linguistics on the other.
Among the outcome measures we have looked for here are recall, satisfaction
and compliance (see Chapter 1).

The studies of Balint (1957) and his colleagues on the doctor–patient
relationships in general practice take place within a different field of beliefs and
practices—that of dynamic psychology. The revolutionary phase of this sort of
research began with the startling formulations of Freud. Here, unconsciously
motivated behaviour is believed to have its sources in earlier experience: the
language of patient and doctor expresses hidden messages whose decoding is a
part of the healing process. Outcome measures here are more elusive, though

some would describe the hoped for insights and self-discoveries as another sort of compliance.

In contrast the sociologist who looks at the doctor–patient relationship is often concerned with issues of power and control, and much of the literature from sociology is shot through with different moral imperatives from those which inform psychological analysis. Here the relationship between doctor and patient is taken as a special case for exploring the relationships between the social classes: the consultation is transformed into a political exegesis. More fundamental still, and underlying many of the value judgements made by consultation researchers, is the belief that the more autonomy the patient can be granted, or can win, the more satisfactory or effective will be the encounter. It is assumed to be good for the patient, and morally uplifting for the doctor, that the patient should endure as much autonomy as his intellect, medical condition and social situation permit. The outcomes here are measured in terms of dominance and submission: the doctor–patient encounter is a contest, with winner and loser.

It may be worth bearing in mind the following observations about normal science, as it relates to studies of the consultation and as it relates to the teaching of doctors. Medicine is a secondary or derivative science, and its practice in part dependent on work carried out in a number of what Kuhn calls primary paradigms—for example biochemistry, genetics, learning theory, atomic physics and so on. These different ways of viewing the same medical task create no dissonance in the medical profession.

In the medical dialogues about diseases, the discussion will be centred on the validity and reliability of experiments, on the confidence that can be placed in the results and on the possibilities of utilizing them. The value judgements which underpin the research come in for scant attention.

Whenever we discuss our teaching about the consultation, or our consultation research, it is unusual for us to debate whether autonomy for the patient is desirable or undesirable. Personal autonomy is held to be both politically and morally acceptable, just as it is in other relationships which have been studied by social and behavioural scientists—for example the marital relationship, where reciprocity and negotiation are believed to be more rewarding for the participants than authority and submission. There is a danger here that the medical consultation may be viewed by both researchers and teachers as simply a special case of other forms of human encounter and relationship. This may be a convenient way of researching and teaching about the consultation, but it may prevent us from posing difficult questions about the intentions of the consultation, which extend beyond the solving of clinically understood puzzles.

It is a basic assumption that the consultation is the vehicle for making decisions about clinical problems. In general practice the doctor is enjoined to compose his diagnoses "simultaneously in physical, psychological and social terms". This broadens the concept of "what is wrong?", to include more than diseases. However, a traditional medical education still presents the feelings of the patient and the social context of the patient and his problem as modifications or explanations or illuminations of pathological processes. Even psychiatry, which for the most part deals with disordered behaviours and perceptions which cannot be correlated with physical changes, nonetheless uses a language and imagery which is essentially mechanistic. These assumptions underpin our thinking about the consultation. When the consultation works well, the doctor quickly uncovers "what is wrong". This wrongness, this medical condition, is seen as having an independent existence before and after the consultation. "What is wrong" is not seen to be intrinsic to the fabric of the consultation, nor is it thought to be modified by the consultation except in terms of speed of discovery or success in management. I will return to this later.

Osler's dictum "Listen to the patient. He is telling you the diagnosis". remains the basis of much that we teach our medical students. We teach that taking the patient's history is the most important part of medical diagnosis, and that all the other clinical acts—the physical examination and laboratory investigations—are relatively unimportant in coming to an understanding of what is wrong. And yet, as Fouceault (1973) points out, the modern medical dialogue began not with a new concern for the patient's subjective experience of the illness, but on the contrary with the 18th century exploration of the patient's silent and interior surfaces. It was the discoveries of pathology, first gross morbid anatomy and later histology, which shaped the clinical dialogue. Later with Laennec's invention of the stethoscope, the interior surfaces began to be observed in much the way that Sydenham, two centuries earlier, had described diseases in terms of their external appearance.

Reiser (1978) provides a fascinating reinterpretation of the development of clinical problem-solving which suggests that the Oslerian precept about listening to the patient may be fundamentally misleading. Reiser says that the content of a modern medical history stems not from a preoccupation with the patient's subjective feelings, but rather from a preoccupation with the physical examination. Far from listening to the patient, the modern clinician is trained to conduct the patient through a fairly rigorous schedule of questions which makes quite clear which aspects of the patient's perceptions are valuable in the solving of medical puzzles, and which are to be rejected as lying outside the medical domain. We teach that the main purpose of the physical examination is to discover data which tend to support or deny the hypothesis which we have made from our history. But this is a half-truth. We deceive ourselves because the history is simply a verbal rehearsal of the physical examination. What we add to this history by way of psycho-social variables may therefore be limited, far more than we are aware, by the preoccupations of a medical history which is conceived as a questionnaire, a schedule that adumbrates the physical examination which is to follow.

So what are our intentions? In this section I have suggested that they are confused for the following reasons. First, each behavioural scientist brings to his exegesis his own preoccupations and his own tools for analysis. Secondly, the medical teachers themselves feel ambiguously about the contribution of the behavioural scientists. However enlightened, we doctors remain captured by the primacy of the disease model, not least because it has been the most powerful we have ever had to explain what is wrong with our patients, and to guide us in our management. We may be aware that the behavioural scientist has more to offer than his comments on our "bedside manner", but in the end we believe that these psycho-social variables have a value which must be related to the accurate detection and management of diseases. If we fail to detect a disease, which is another way of saying that the disease model does not help us in this particular instance, what then is the value of the consultation? By what will we judge the consultation's accuracy or effectiveness? It is all very well to exhibit a sensitivity to the patient's mood, to negotiate the relationship, to reassure appropriately, or to instruct concisely and clearly—but to what end if "what is wrong?" does not lie securely within the domain of our clinical understanding. At the very least, when we behave in a way which might be approved by the behavioural scientist, within a consultation where the disease model does not succeed, how do we differ from the social worker or the lawyer or the friend? We doctors cannot look to our behavioural science colleagues for an answer to these questions, because they too have taken our medicine at its face value. Attempts to coin a new phrase, or invent a new profession like "clinical sociology" (Glassner and Freeman, 1979), hardly address the issues.

Lastly, we may be faltering because we have become too ambitious. The term "disease" refers to a whole spectrum of different concepts, which are importantly and profoundly different from one another not only phenomenologically, but in terms of the history of the ideas which they embody. The description of heart disease in terms of specific heart valve deformities was paramount when the end-point of these diseases was early death from heart failure and confirmation at post-mortem. With the invention of specific and powerful remedies for heart failure, remedies which could be applied independently of the valvular lesions which caused the cardiac embarrassment, physiological rather than anatomical descriptions of diseases became paramount: one talked of a decompensated left-ventricular failure, rather than of an anatomical description of what caused that failure. Now with the signal success of open-heart surgery, the valvular diagnosis again becomes important, an accurate description vital to the outcome. Gout, streptococcal arthritis and a tear of the internal meniscus, may all result in a painful knee, but as ideas embrace totally separate concepts of "disease". The differentiation of these ideas, their history and their underlying assumptions, constitute the core of medical teaching and research.

We have not yet looked at the consultation in this way. We may have a quite false expectation that all consultations can be understood by the application of one embracing model. Of course the everyday experience of general practitioners suggests that this is not so. We have done little to describe what we experience, and less still to build a theoretical infrastructure. Again Balint and his colleagues have made a beginning. In "Six Minutes for the Patient" (Balint and Norell, 1974) and "Treatment or Diagnosis: a study of repeat prescriptions in general practice" (Balint *et al.*, 1970), some attempt was made to look at a particular sort of clinical encounter and to speculate on its meaning.

4 WHAT IS THE DIRECTION IN WHICH WE ARE LIKELY TO MOVE?

Speculation in print is always a risky business. For this reason alone, I will limit myself to the graduate training of the general practitioner and to general practice-based research.

The growing recognition that continuing medical education for general practice was based on the same inappropriate assumptions as his previous pregraduate education has led to an interest in performance review (Working Party of the Royal College of General Practitioners, 1981). At first it was thought that evidence about performance review could only be reliably achieved by epidemiological methods. In this sense performance review would become yet another mode, albeit a local and unambitious one, of health services research. But this research in general practice has tended to limit the imagination of the research worker, and to predict that the variables which he will measure will be those which now preoccupy health services researchers in community medicine. We have therefore a growing literature which examines the workload, morbidity, prescriptions and the like, which can then be expressed in terms of the structure of the health service, or the demographic descriptions of the patients. The methodology is a respectable one, and the conclusions which it reaches can be expressed in reliable terms of likelihood. Unfortunately, because the variables tend to be so limited, the questions to which this research addresses itself become increasingly banal and the answers increasingly predictable.

More recently an attempt has been made to evaluate the general practitioner's work holistically, much in the way in which the general practitioner proposes to look at his patient. Central to this activity, it has been suggested that the consultations themselves, prerecorded on videotape, should be subject to an evaluation. There have been a number of attempts to construct an evaluation grid for all consultations. My own favourite one, which incidentally is most likely to be widely tried at the moment, is the Pendleton *et al.* (in press) schedule. This demands that the consultation be evaluated in relation to a number of different aspects of the doctor's work. Each one of them is of course a value judgement—though, in the case of Pendleton *et al.*, this judgement was negotiated with many groups of doctors looking at their own consultation video-tapes, over a number of years. And in relation to each of these "judgements", the individual evaluators are invited to make their own assessments about success or failure.

The natural scientist must shrink in horror from such goings-on. What is the validity of the variables being measured? What can reliability between observers mean, other than some form of mutual brainwashing which will result in them all responding with Pavlovian predictability to a particular set of signals from the television screen?

In part the answer lies in the nature of medicine, and its difference, its separateness from science. Munson (1981) argues that unlike biology, medicine is an enterprise in which all activities must be subservient to the urgent task of healing patients and curing diseases. It is by these criteria, and not by the impeccable rules of pure scientific investigation, that medicine judges itself and is judged by society. Its internal aims are concerned first not with knowledge, but with responding maximally to the needs of the patient. This is not to say that much of medicine cannot be reduced, in terms of research, to the activities of the biological or behavioural scientist. But it cannot, and in practice it never is, limited by them.

What will emerge from the use of instruments like the Pendleton *et al.* (in press) schedule are not so much answers as a new way of framing questions. From this I believe will grow a different sort of research which will parallel that concerned with what behavioural scientists now measure—compliance, recall, dominance, role and the like. In terms of pure science, this research may be even more disreputable than the evaluation of consultations for performance review. It will, I think, be essentially phenomenological, it will concentrate on every aspect of the consultation as narrative, drama, communication and, of course, problem-solving. I say problem-solving here, rather than puzzle-solving. The reforming zeal of Laurence Weed (1969) in adapting the medical record for better clinical care, teaching and research, was concerned with the solving not of problems, whose nature cannot be predicted, but of puzzles (that is to say diseases or personal crises) whose nature is predicated by the assumptive world of the teaching hospital.

The shift to performance review in continuing medical education for general practice, particularly that important aspect concerned with an evaluation of consultations, may give fresh impetus to a more open and explorative form of research in general practice than before, because traditional medical education simply reinforces a preoccupation with models and variables which have in the past proved useful.

If doctors are encouraged in large numbers to contemplate the video-recording of their own clinical work, to see time and again not simply the strength of the conventional disease model but its limitations, and I would add also to see the strength and limitations of the conventional behavioural science models, the search will be on for other conceptual tools which may guide us in the care of patients.

Two studies in which I have myself been involved, concerning patients on repeat prescriptions and women who come to hysterectomy, lead me to believe that we will begin by exploring not explicative models but managerial ones. These latter already exist in profusion in general practice, but we cannot discern their shape because we have been taught to ignore them.

One further concept may be helpful in all this. Elsewhere I have suggested (Marinker, in press) that contemporary general practice in the U.K., the U.S.A. and similar developed countries, seeks in its rhetoric to respond to the highest levels of Maslow's hierarchy of needs (Maslow, 1968). We represent the medicine of extreme affluence, and the definitions of health which we recognize approximate to Maslow's highest goal of self-actualization. But not all consultations are concerned with this level of need. Part of the negotiation which takes place between doctor and patient may therefore be concerned, albeit unconsciously, with a decision about hierarchical levels. The treatment of scabies may not be directly concerned with self-actualization: but the request to go on the pill by a 42-year-old wife of a man who was sterilized at her request, is clearly concerned with a whole spectrum of upper-level hierarchies, as well as with many basic ones.

Morris (1972) turns to the theatre to provide another model of human encounters: routines, rituals and dramas. In my own teaching (Marinker, 1981) I invite medical students and trainees to attempt a similar classification of consultations.

Type I consultations are *Routines*. Usually both the situation and the patient are familiar to the general practitioner, and the type of problem is a common one. A three-year-old child is brought into the surgery and the mother explains that she has been crying all night. The child looks hot, has a nasal discharge, and the doctor makes an "educated guess" that the child is suffering an infection of the middle ear. Otitis media is far and away the most likely explanation of this presentation and the general practitioner will test this by examining the ear drums.

Type II consultations are *Rituals*. Here the clinical content of the consultation may be hard to discern. Usually a repeat prescription is issued because of some disease or some unexplained symptoms which were first dealt with in the past, sometimes years in the past. The repeat prescription has a psychological or symbolic significance for the patient, long after it ceases to have any pharmacological intention. In this sort of consultation there seems to be no attempt to solve a problem, but rather to reaffirm a relationship, albeit not a very close one.

Type III consultations are *Dramas*. Morris judges an encounter as being dramatic when it fulfils the following three criteria. First, the situation must be novel within the person's experience. He goes on to say that this does not mean that every aspect of it must be quite unfamiliar, but that important aspects of it are new. Secondly, the activity, or its outcome, must be important. Thirdly, the outcome must be in doubt.

In Type III consultations the problems which are presented to the doctor may be novel or presented in a novel way. Both the activity of the problem-solving and the outcome for the patient, are important and uncertain. An obese woman of 50 presents with double vision and an obvious squint. The diagnosis of diabetes mellitus with a neuropathy of the sixth cranial nerve will not come readily as an informed guess. There is no familiar pattern to be recognized from the fragments of what the patient presents.

One may speculate that consultations become dysfunctional when doctor and patient fail to negotiate about or recognize the dramatic status of the encounter.

The role of the healer predates by millennia the discoveries of contemporary biotechnology. The literature of general practice describes the unintended consequences of our technical preoccupations: not only the technical pre-occupations of the profession, but the technical expectations of the patients who consult us. In both human and economic terms, it is one of the sharpest challenges to general practice to determine those situations in which the application of this technology should be applied or withheld. The earlier functions of medicine, to reassure, to legitimate, to celebrate, to propitiate, to discipline, to share suffering—all these are still discernible on our contemporary video-screens. In building future tools for assessment, models for understanding the consultation, we may need to develop not only a sense of the politics of the consultation, but of its archaeology.

5 HOW WILL DOCTORS AND BEHAVIOURAL SCIENTISTS RELATE?

The earlier chapters in this book are testimony to a vigorous and growing relationship. In the future we should be prepared for a whole spectrum of such relationships.

First, we should be prepared for and welcome an adversarial relationship.

The critique mounted by the social scientist on the behaviour of the doctor in the consultation has demanded a certain distance between the two professions, a willingness to apply the assumptions and tools of one profession to an examination of the assumptions and tools of another, without the danger of contamination or collusion. This sort of work which we do together in the pursuit of a more effective and humane medicine will remain important. But the quality of that work will depend not only on a willingness by the medical profession to open itself up to such critical gaze. It will depend also on the sensitivity of the behavioural scientist to the medical context of what he sees, and perhaps most of all on the ability of the behavioural scientist to develop a more penetrating and appropriate analysis of human interaction.

There remains also the possibility of a new convergent line of development, in which the intention must be a true contamination of one discipline with the other, and in this I include a contamination of the ideas of one behavioural scientist with the other behavioural scientists. The research which may result from such a convergence will no doubt have its roots in the Balint researches of ten and 20 years ago, in the grounded theory approach of Goffman (1971), and it may borrow much from such fields as archaeological, historical and literary research.

6 WHAT WILL BE THE EFFECTS OF ALL THIS?

This book suggests that the consultation itself, as an event or series of events in its own right, is coming to be seen in a new light. Throughout my own education at medical school and beyond, I saw the consultation as the necessary encounter without which the *real task* of medicine, the diagnosis and treatment of disease, could not be carried out. But what if there were other *real tasks* in medicine. What if the encounter itself came to be seen, using the language of Donabedian (1967), not as a process but as an outcome? If the consultation then can be at one and the same time a process in the sense that it is concerned with the diagnosis and management of a clinical problem, and an outcome in that it represents an end in itself, the definitive answer to the question that it poses, we will require new forms of analysis and new criteria for judgement. Such a quantum jump in thinking is unlikely to be achieved in the cosy confines of, say general practice or social psychology. But it may come from the confusion and perhaps even the fusion of both. That may be the distant prize for patient care which we start to win now when we teach about the consultation, when we puzzle over the communication, and when we try to measure its dimensions and to interpret what it is that we are about.

REFERENCES

Balint, M. (1957). *The Doctor, His Patient and The Illness.* Pitman, London.
Balint, E. and Norell, J. S. (1974). *Six Minutes for the Patient.* Tavistock Publications, London.
Balint, M., Hunt, J., Joyce, D., Marinker, M. and Woodcock, J. (1970). *Treatment and Diagnosis: A Study of Repeat Prescriptions in General Practice.* Tavistock Publications, London.
Donabedian, A. (1967). Evaluating the quality of medical care. *Milbank Memorial Fund Quarterly,* 44 part 2, 166–206.
Fouceault, M. (1973). *The Birth of the Clinic.* Tavistock Publications, London.
Glassner and Freedman (1979). *Clinical Sociology.* Longman, New York.
Goffman, E. (1971). *Relations in Public.* Allen Lane, Harmondsworth.
Kuhn, T. (1962). *The Structure of Scientific Revolutions.* Chicago University Press, Chicago.
Marinker, M. (1981). *'Clinical Method' in Teaching General Practice.* Klurver-Medical, London.
Marinker, M. (in press). A climate of opinion. *A Symposium on the Family in Medicine.* University of Michigan Medical School, Michigan.
Mazlo, A. H. (1968). *Towards a Psychology of Being.* Van Nostrand, New York.
Morris, J. (1972). In *Six Approaches to the Person,* (R. Ruddock, ed.). Routledge and Kegan Paul, London.
Munson, R. (1981). Why medicine cannot be a science. *J. Med. Phil.* 6, 183.
Pendleton, D. A., Schofield, T. P. C., Tate, P. H. L. and Havelock, P. B. (in press). *The Consultation: An Approach to Learning and Teaching.* Oxford University Press, Oxford.
Reiser, S. J. (1978). The decline of the clinical dialogue. *J. Med. Phil.* 3, 305.
Weed, L. L. (1969). *Medical Records, Medical Education and Patient Care.* Case Western Reserve University Press, Cleveland.
Working Party of the Royal College of General Practitioners (1981). What sort of doctor? *J. Roy. Coll. Gen. Pract.* 31, 232.

Index